Methods for Hematological Analysis in Fish

Methods for Hematological Analysis in Fish

Maria José T. Ranzani-Paiva

Santiago Benites de Pádua

Marcos Tavares-Dias

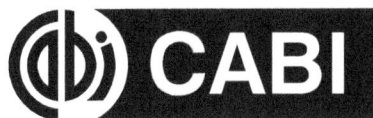

CABI

CABI is a trading name of CAB International

CABI
Nosworthy Way
Wallingford
Oxfordshire OX10 8DE
UK

CABI
200 Portland Street
Boston
MA 02114
USA

Tel: +44 (0)1491 832111
E-mail: info@cabi.org
Website: www.cabi.org

T: +1 (617)682-9015
E-mail: cabi-nao@cabi.org

The views expressed in this publication are those of the author(s) and do not necessarily represent those of, and should not be attributed to, CAB International (CABI). Any images, figures and tables not otherwise attributed are the author(s)' own. References to internet websites (URLs) were accurate at the time of writing.

CAB International and, where different, the copyright owner shall not be liable for technical or other errors or omissions contained herein. The information is supplied without obligation and on the understanding that any person who acts upon it, or otherwise changes their position in reliance thereon, does so entirely at their own risk. Information supplied is neither intended nor implied to be a substitute for professional advice. The reader/user accepts all risks and responsibility for losses, damages, costs and other consequences resulting directly or indirectly from using this information.

CABI's Terms and Conditions, including its full disclaimer, may be found at https://www.cabidigital-library.org/terms-and-conditions.

A catalogue record for this book is available from the British Library, London, UK.

ISBN-13: 9781836991748 (hardback)
9781836991755 (ePDF)
9781836991762 (ePub)

DOI: 10.1079/9781836991762.0000

Commissioning Editor: Jamie Lee
Editorial Assistant: Theresa Regueira
Production Editor: James Bishop

Typeset by Exeter Premedia Services Pvt Ltd, Chennai, India
Printed in the USA

Acknowledgments

The authors thank those who contributed to the production of this work. We are especially grateful to Drs Maria Helena da Silva Pitombeira, Antenor Aguiar Santos, and Ângela Teresa Silva e Souza for their critical analysis of the manuscript; to MSc Wemesson Ferreira for help with cytochemistry; to Márcia Mayumi Ishikawa for help with the cell's photos; and to Márcia Navarro Cipólli for the initial review of the manuscript. We thank Dr A. Leyva for the English translation and editing. We are also thankful to FAPESP for the support (Proc. No. 2013/07289-6).

Summary

Preface   ix

Presentation   xi

Authors biographies   xiii

1 Clinical Hematology of Fish   1
   Circulatory System   1
   Blood   2
   Hematological Techniques   3

2 Collection of Blood   4
   Capture of Fish   4
   Confinement of Fish   4
   Anticoagulants   6
   Circulatory System of Fish   7
   Puncture of Blood Vessels or Heart   7
   Storage of Blood After Collection   12

3 Hemogram   14
   Part 1: Erythrogram   14
   Red Blood Cell Counting (RBC)   14
   Hematocrit   20
   Hemoglobin Concentration   22
   Calculation of RBC indices   23

4 Hemogram   28
   Part II: White Blood Count (WBC) and Thrombocyte Count (THRC)   28
   Blood Smear Staining   29
   Total White Blood Cells   32
   White Blood Cell Differential or Formula   32
   Interpretation of WBC Count   34
   Thrombocytes and Erythroblasts   34
   Morpho-Physiological Description of Blood Cells of Fish   34
   Study of Blood Parasites   42

5   Cytochemical Methods Used for Blood Cells   **51**
Periodic Acid-Schiff Method   52
Phosphatases   52
Method for Alkaline Phosphatase   54
Method for Acid Phosphatase   56
Method for Peroxidase (Myeloperoxidase)   57
Method for Non-Specific Esterase   59
Blue Precipitate in the Cytoplasm of Leukocytes   60
Sudan Black B Method   60
Bromophenol Blue Method   61
Metachromatic Staining   62

References   **69**

Annex 1   **77**

Index   **79**

Preface

I thank Dr Maria José Tavares Ranzani-Paiva for graciously giving me the honor of writing the foreword to this book, "Methods for hematological analysis in fish," which is now available to the public. This was a well-known dream of this renowned hematologist, which has become a reality through the collaboration of three competent researchers.

As explained in Chapter I, sensing the inadequacy of many adapted methods from veterinary clinical hematology of domestic mammals, the authors proposed to provide a book that would make it possible to standardize the protocols used in fish hematology. Thus, Chapter II presents the most appropriate precautions and techniques, from the capture and anesthesia of the fish for the collection of blood samples, in a clear and objective way.

In the following chapters, the authors present, in an interesting and detailed way, the makeup of the complete blood count, its analyses and interpretations, bringing theory to practice. The morphological description of the blood cells of fish of different species is presented in a comparative manner and with rich illustrations.

Finally, Chapter V discusses the cytochemical methods applied in blood cell studies, combining the techniques for practicality and importance.

Throughout the book, there is absolute discretion and firm purpose in teaching and clarifying complex issues of fish hematology, making it within the reach of all in a simple and clear language. With the certainty of success as a contribution of great value in the guidance and scientific training of new professionals, I compliment the authors for such an impressive work.

Ângela Teresa Silva e Souza

Presentation

The aim of this book was to standardize the protocols used in hematological procedures for fish studies, which have been used by researchers all over the world. It is the result of several years of research and is part of the Aquabrasil Project Component Health Status of Cultivated Aquatic Organisms (PC Sanidade), conceived with the objective of promoting the technological leap of Brazilian aquaculture, which began at the end of 2007.

In Chapter I, the protocols used in fish hematology are described, and a standard is established so that all the research results obtained in this area can be better presented and discussed.

Chapter II demonstrates and discusses the most appropriate care and techniques, from capture and anesthesia to the collection of blood samples in a clear and objective way, so that beginners and hematology researchers can have no doubts.

In the following two chapters, the makeup of the blood cell count and its analysis and interpretation are presented and worked out in detail, bringing the supporting theory to practice. The morphological description of the blood cells of fish of different species is presented comparatively and with rich illustrations. Finally, Chapter V discusses cytochemical methods applied in blood cell studies, combining the techniques for their practicality and importance.

This work is the first of its kind in Brazil that arises from the wishes of the authors to elucidate some of the basic and inherent issues in the hematological investigation of fish. However, there are still many doubts to be resolved and we hope that this will serve as a support for the studies of the fish blood and that such studies will be more frequent and enlightening.

Authors biographies

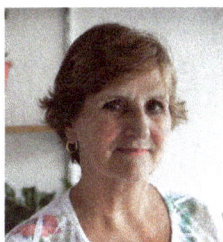

Maria José Tavares Ranzani-Paiva
BS in biology from the University of Brasilia (1972) and PhD in ecology and natural resources from the Federal University of São Carlos (1993), Brazil. She is a retired scientific researcher VI from the Fisheries Institute of Brazil and CNPq IC researcher. In 1997, she completed post-doctoral training at the University of Porto, Portugal, with the support of FAPESP.

She served as director of the aquatic fisheries division of the Fisheries Institute (1993-1995), editor of the Boletim do Instituto de Pesca (Fisheries Institute Bulletin) (1996-2001), president of the Brazilian Association of Pathologists of Aquatic Organisms (ABRAPOA) (1992-1994), and vice post-graduation coordinator in aquaculture and fisheries of the Fisheries Institute (2004-2007). She was a coordinator of the agricultural sciences area of FAPESP from 2007 to 2019. Since 2001, she has been a supervisor of the aquaculture post-graduation course at the Aquaculture Center of UNESP and, since 2004, of the post-graduate program in aquaculture and fisheries of the Fisheries Institute. She has published about 130 scientific articles in the areas of hematology of aquatic organisms, parasitology, aquatic toxicology, nutrition, fish farming, frog farming, and others. Besides, she has organized two books: *Health of Aquatic Organisms and Technology* and *Aquatic Organisms*.

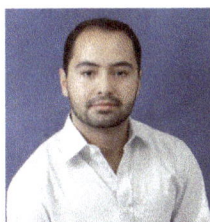

Santiago Benites de Pádua
He graduated in veterinary medicine from Faculty of Anhanguera de Dourados (2010), MS in aquaculture from the Aquaculture Center of Paulista State University (2013), Estate of São Paulo, Brazil. He is a researcher at the Fisheries Laboratory of Embrapa Agropecuária Oeste and the Laboratory of Pathology of Aquatic Organisms of the Aquaculture Center of UNESP. He has published dozens of scientific articles in the areas of clinical hematology, parasitology, and fish bacteriology, as well as book chapters dealing with fish hematology. He is a founding partner of AquiVet Saúde Aquática, where he acts in the implementation of disease control and eradication programs in nursery farms producing fingerlings.

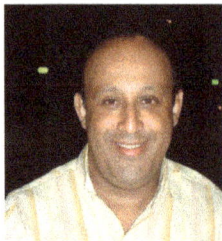

Marcos Tavares-Dias

He is a biologist, graduated from Uni-Mauá of Ribeirão Preto (1989), PhD in aquaculture of continental waters from the UNESP Jaboticabal Aquaculture Center (2003), São Paulo, Brazil. He was a professor and researcher at the Federal University of Amazonas (2004-2008). He is a member of the Brazilian Association of Pathologists of Aquatic Organisms (ABRAPOA). Currently, he works as a scientific researcher at Embrapa Amapá, Pará, Brazil, and is a PQ/CNPq researcher. He has served as an adviser in the post-graduate course in tropical biodiversity at the Federal University of Amapá since 2008, and in the post-graduate program Rede Bionorte at the Federal University of Amazonas since 2010. He has published about 90 scientific articles in the areas of fish hematology and chelonian, parasitology, pisciculture, toxicology, and fish treatment. In addition, he has authored seven book chapters and technical works. He also published a book on fish hematology and organized a book on fish health and aquaculture.

1 Clinical Hematology of Fish

Hematology is the study of blood, or the sum of our knowledge of blood. Much of this information consists of measurements of hematological parameters under normal and abnormal conditions. The application of hematological studies in animal research and disease processes in humans is well accepted and considered a routine procedure in diagnostic methods. Detailed comparative studies of man and domestic animals have provided conditions for assuming that blood is one of the 'mirrors' that reflects the vital processes that take place in organisms.

With the intensification of fish production, health problems have become more frequent, making it necessary to periodically monitor the health conditions of fish in a breeding environment. In this scenario, clinical hematology plays an essential role, acting as a tool that allows the evaluation of the defense conditions of an animal and allows the researcher and breeder to identify the responses of fish to the challenges of breeding in an effective manner and without resorting to expensive resources.

Among the main challenges to which fish are constantly exposed in breeding conditions are population densities; occurrence of endo- and ectoparasites; exposure to bacteria, fungi, and potentially pathogenic viruses; alteration of environmental quality conditions, such as physical and chemical variables of nursery waters; presence of toxic agents; damage caused by inadequate periodic management and unbalanced diet. All these conditions determine a series of changes in the blood constituents studied. However, these hematological responses are differential, showing peculiarities related to the stimuli to which the fish are subjected, and the differences related to the various species bred and to their biology and ecological habits.

Thus, when establishing reference values, these peculiarities should be considered, in the same way that additional studies should be conducted to characterize fish responses to other challenges.

Circulatory System

Most body organs have some degree of independence, though they are related to one another and important for the functioning of the body as a whole. The circulatory system, on the other hand, extends throughout the animal's body and is interconnected with all other tissues, through which the blood carries the substances indispensable to the maintenance of the vital processes of each cell. Functionally, the blood vessels irrigate all the body tissues, except the epithelial and cartilaginous ones. Due to this physiological condition, the study of blood becomes strategic for evaluating homeostasis in fish. In this study, several researchers have used clinical hematology, among other tools, as a method to evaluate nutritional requirements, such as requirements of minerals for Nile tilapia (Oreochromis niloticus) (Barros *et al.*, 2002; Ferrari *et al.*, 2004; Hisano *et al.*, 2007), of vitamins for pirarucu (*Arapaima gigas*) (Andrade *et al.*, 2007) and 'matrinxã' (*Brycon amazonicus*) (Affonso *et al.*, 2007), *Carassius auratus*, Oreochromis niloticus, and. The hematological parameters have also been used in the evaluation of the deleterious effects of pesticides in ichthyotoxicology, such as those performed in Nile tilapia (Sweilum, 2006; El-Sayed *et al.*, 2007), jundiá (*Rhamdia quelen*) (Crestani *et al.*, 2006; Melo *et al.*, 2006; Borges *et al.*, 2007), *Labeo rohita* (Das and Mukherjee, 2003; Adhikari *et al.*, 2004), and tilapia, besides studies on health, mainly involving parasites

DOI: 10.1079/9781836991762.0001

(Martins et al., 2004; Ranzani-Paiva et al., 2005; Ghiraldelli et al., 2006; Tavares-Dias et al., 2007a; Biller et al., 2022; Wang et al., 2021) and bacteria (Ranzani-Paiva et al., 2004; Martins et al., 2008 a, b; Garcia and Moraes, 2009; Yu et al., 2010).

The blood count can also be used as a diagnostic method, especially when it comes to hemoparasitosis. Up to now, the presence of hemoflagellates, such as Trypanosoma and Cryptobia, and intracellular parasites as well, such as hemoggregins, have been described. In addition to these, rickettsial agents have recently been described to parasitize blood monocytes of the hybrid surubim (*Pseudoplatystoma reticulatum × P. corruscans*).

The study of fish blood constituents can even be used as a prognostic indicator of pathological conditions, especially when considering morphological changes in blood cells. These evaluations allow us to identify the different degrees of response of fish when diseased, in which the severity of the changes implies a worse condition when challenged. In this sense, Satake et al. (2009) described the main morphological changes observed in the blood cells of teleost fish under breeding. In addition, the etiopathogenesis of diseases can be obtained through hematological evaluation in both quantitative and qualitative parameters.

Blood

Blood is a liquid tissue, mobile and in balance with virtually all other tissues, and it has interstitial substances that are great homeostatic forces of the animal. It distributes heat, transports respiratory gases, nutrients, degraded products, and flows through specialized sensory tissues, capable of selectively reacting to factors such as osmotic pressure, pH, temperature, and levels of certain hormones.

Information on the status of the animal is obtained by studying the blood through physiological, biochemical, and other methods. Together with the determination of the number of indicators of the liquid part of the blood

(plasma and serum), the study of its morphology also plays an important role in hematology. In fish, as in other vertebrates, the presence, amount, and proportion of the different cells in the peripheral (vascular) blood reflect a specific physiological state of the animal at a given time during a certain period of life. In other words, the composition, proportion, and amount of the standard elements in the blood are closely related to the functional state of the fish.

Fish have developed numerous adaptive strategies to ensure their survival in the aquatic environment, where extreme variations in temperature, salinity, pressure, pH, O_2, and CO_2 occur. These adaptations include (1) development of a large proportion of red muscles and increase of the gill surface to facilitate aerobic metabolism in waters with low O_2 concentration; (2) development of air breathing in some; (3) seasonal movements for sites with higher O_2 concentrations; and (4) development of heterogeneous hemoglobin as a possible mechanism of adaptation to the unstable environment.

Fish also have the ability to use different organs to form blood cells when the main organ is affected, for example, by some diseases. Therefore, it is difficult to characterize the leukocyte picture of fish with lesions in the liver, kidney, spleen, and so on. Due to all these factors, the morphological picture of fish blood is complicated and difficult to standardize.

There is qualitative and quantitative morphological variation of the blood components of fish, in the face of endogenous conditions, such as sex, stage of gonadal maturation, weight, length, nutritional status, intense muscular activity, or diseases (Ranzani-Paiva, 1995a,b; Steinhagen et al., 1997; Gabriel et al., 2004; Ranzani-Paiva et al., 2005; Barros et al., 2009; Santos et al., 2009; Hrubec et al., 2010; Yu et al., 2010; Seriani et al., 2010a, b; Tavares-Dias et al., 2011; Seriani and Ranzani-Paiva, 2012), or exogenous conditions, such as temperature, O_2 and CO_2 concentration in the water, seasonal cycle, stress, pollutants, and so on (Barcelos et al., 2004; Gabriel et al., 2004; Kirschbaum et al., 2009; Santos et al., 2009; Stoskopf, 2010; Jerônimo et al., 2011; Seriani et al., 2011). The last ones are also related to the type of environment in which the fish lives.

Hematological Techniques

The simplicity of most blood sampling techniques is probably responsible for the growing increase in the use of hematology as a means of establishing the health status of fish.

Although clinical hematology is of great importance in fish production systems and in laboratories for the clinical evaluation of animals, some techniques routinely employed until now have not been standardized. The protocols adopted in veterinary clinical hematology of domestic mammals are used to a large extent in fish procedures, but the techniques used white blood cell and thrombocyte counts are not adequate (Tavares-Dias et al., 2002; Ishikawa et al., 2008). These same difficulties are shared in the hematology of other non-mammalian vertebrates, the so-called pirenematas animals (which have permanently nucleated erythrocytes). Thus, some differentiated methods have been established to address this shortcoming and will be discussed in Chapters IV and V. In addition, the identification of blood cells in different species of fish has been controversial. These imperfections have already been described by other investigators, especially Tavares-Dias and Moraes (2004).

Hematological techniques are used in three ways in the following order:

- differentiation of normal from abnormal blood;
- diagnosis of disease or abnormality; and
- detailed hematological studies.

With blood samples, it is possible to do hematological, bacteriological, parasitological, biochemical, toxicological, and serological tests and blood typing for transfusion (not the case for fish). Accordingly, hematology is of importance as a physiological analysis and is an aid in the diagnosis of diseases. Blood tests can determine the severity of the condition and evaluate response to treatment. In addition, the morphological changes in cells are useful in toxicological analyses, such as the appearance of micronuclei, besides being important as a follow-up study. In this context, hematological analyses in fish exposed to contaminants may be emerging to monitor environmental quality. Several authors have already described changes in some blood components associated with exposure to environmental pollutants and their prospects for use in monitoring aquatic ecosystems, and these studies have contributed to understanding the toxic effects of contaminants released into water bodies (Ranzani-Paiva and Silva-Souza, 2004; Tavares-Dias and Moraes, 2004; Seriani et al., 2011, 2012).

The aim of this book was to standardize protocols used in hematological procedures for fish studies, which have been used by researchers all over Brazil.

It is the result of several years of research by the authors and, in addition, it is part of the Aquabrasil Project Component: Health Status of Cultivated Organisms (PC Health), designed to promote the technological leap of Brazilian aquaculture, which began at the end of 2007.

2 Collection of Blood

For a more accurate hematological examination, blood collection procedures should be performed quickly and without causing additional stress to the fish, since capture and mechanical containment, when performed inappropriately, cause a series of changes in hematological parameters of fish, as a secondary response to the stress stimulus. Thus, this chapter describes the basic procedures that must be followed to succeed in collecting blood from fish.

Capture of Fish

The animals must be taken from the river, sea, lake, nursery, or tank with the aid of a net or hand net. It is not necessary to make the total collection of blood from all specimens. Generally, this is done with a sample, which can be two, five, ten, or as many specimens as required for the work. Table 2.1 shows the fish numbers for sampling, according to the desired confidence level and the number of animals in the population, for a statistically representative evaluation. However, this number cannot always be obtained in practice. What is recommended is that sampling be as large as possible without loss of quality. This is common sense. The sampling may be from healthy or diseased fish, depending on the purpose of the study. The fish should be caught considering adequate conditions of both the environment and the animal, that is, water temperature not too low and fish fasting for at least 12 hour.

In studies of free-living populations, animals should be captured in the most appropriate manner, both for the fish and for the purpose of the study, respecting the animals' welfare. For example, the use of a hold-net or trawl-net is not recommended for hematological studies, since they cause severe animal injuries. If possible, always use the same procedures from the beginning to the end of the study. The number of animals collected in the natural environment will also depend on the objectives of the work and the success of capture. What is recommended in this case is that the sample be more than 30. Stress to the animal should be minimized, and care must be taken so that there is no excessive loss of mucus.

All such care is necessary if animals are to be reintroduced into the breeding or natural environment after collection of blood, with a lower risk of death, and for the preservation of the material to be examined.

Confinement of Fish

For the appropriate collection of blood, the fish should be properly contained, preferably with a damp cloth over the eyes. The use of an anesthetic is recommended to reduce or mitigate stress in fish, but its use may also cause hematological changes; therefore, anesthetics are used with some restrictions and at the dose indicated for each species and age (Table 2.2). Any and all blood collection procedures require the operator's competence and speed to be efficient and cause minimal injury to the fish.

Several anesthetics are used for blood collection procedures in fish: chlorobutanol, benzocaine, clove oil and its derivatives (eugenol, isoeugenol, and methyleugenol), menthol, MS 222, and 2-phenoxyethanol (Inoue et al., 2004). Some of them are listed below with the protocol for their use.

Chlorobutanol
Chlorobutanol .... 50.0 g
70% ethanol .... 1,000.0 mL

Methods for Haematological Analysis in Fish (Maria José Ranzani Paiva *et al.*)
DOI: 10.1079/9781836991762.0002

Table 2.1. Number of specimens to be analyzed according to statistical reliability and population size (Moriñigo, personal communication). (Table author's own.)

	Population size									
P	100	500	1000	5000	10,000	25,000	50,000	100,000	500,000	1×10^6
0.1%	–	–	950	2253	2587	2822	2906	2950	2985	2990
0.5%	–	349	450	563	580	591	595	596	597	598
1%	95	224	258	289	294	295	296	296	296	296
10%	25	28	28	28	28	28	28	28	30	30

Table 2.2. Hematological changes in fish probably caused by the use of anesthetic. (Table author's own.)

Anesthetic	Species	Changes	Author
Benzocaine	Oreochromis niloticus	Increased hematocrit	Delbon (2006)
Benzocaine	Urophycis brasiliensis	Increased number of erythrocytes and hemoglobin rate	Bolsaína (2006)
Clove oil	Oncorhynchus mykiss	Increased erythrocyte number and decreased MCHC	Tort et al. (2002)
Eugenol	Oreochromis niloticus	Decreased RBC, hematocrit, and changes in indexeshematimetric	Delbon (2010)
Eugenol	Colossoma macropomum	Increased hematocrit	Inoue et al. (2011)
Powdered cloves	Huso huso	RBC increase, hemoglobin, hematocrit and changes in hematimetric indices	Mohammadiaraejabad et al. (2009)
Powdered cloves	Rutilus rutilus	RBC increase, hemoglobin, hematocrit and changes in hematimetric indices	Sudagar et al. (2009)
2-phenoxyethanol	Sparus aurata	Increased erythrocyte number, hematocrit, and increased MCHC	Tort et al. (2002)
2-phenoxyethanol	Cyprinus carpio	Increase in hematocrit levels and percentage of monocytes	Velíšek et al. (2007a)
2-phenoxyethanol	Silurus glanis	Increased levels of hematocrit, MCV, and MCHC	Velíšek et al. (2007b)

If there is difficulty with dissolving, add acetone, a little at a time with constant mixing. Add 1.0 mL of this solution to 1 L of water. This anesthetic has the disadvantage of being expensive and carcinogenic.

Benzocaine

Benzocaine .... 3.0 g
70% ethanol ....
20.0 mL
Use 3.0 mL of this solution per 1 L of water.

Clove oil

Crude clove oil .... 5.0 mL
96–99% ethanol .... 95.0 mL
Use 1–1.5 mL of this solution per 1 L of water.

Menthol

Menthol crystals...................... 10.0 g
96–99% ethanol .... 90.0 mL
Use 0.5–1.0 mL of this solution per 1 L of water.

It should be noted that the doses of such drugs may be different depending on the species in question, and therefore, the appropriate dose should be confirmed beforehand. For blood collection, the fish should be completely anesthetized (2–5 min). Recovery will occur 5–10 min after removal of the fish from the anesthetic bath, with variations according to the active principle used. For euthanizing the animal, anesthesia needs to be deeper.

Anticoagulants

For a blood count, clotting must be prevented and several anticoagulants are used: oxalates, citrates, EDTA, heparin, and others. Of those, the most commonly used is heparin, an antithrombotic substance, because it is a natural anticoagulant. However, it has the disadvantage of having a high cost. The anticoagulant activity exerted by heparin is promoted by the acceleration of antithrombin III activity, which, in turn, inhibits the action of thrombin and other proteases responsible for the coagulation cascade (Harr *et al.*, 2005).

EDTA is also widely used, which is the only one that prevents the aggregation of thrombocytes. Simply moistening syringes and needles (preferably disposable) with anticoagulant solution prevents clotting when blood is drawn. The choice of anticoagulant should be the one that does not modify the normal characteristics of blood. The anticoagulant volume in the syringe should be minimal so as to avoid dilution. It should be remembered that excess anticoagulant may interfere with the method used, since, in addition to diluting the blood, if only a small amount is collected, it can cause cell lysis and affect leukocyte morphology. Table 2.3 lists some of the hematological changes that can be caused by the use of anticoagulants.

Table 2.3. Hematological changes in fish can be caused by the use of anticoagulants.

Anticoagulant	Species	Changes
EDTA	Five teleosts species	Increased globular volume and hemolysis
Na₂EDTA	*Morone chrysops × M. saxatilis*	Increased hematocrit
Na₂EDTA	*Cyprinus carpio*	Increased osmotic fragility of erythrocytes; changes in the proportion of lymphocytes, increase in reactive O₂ species, anisocytosis, and anisocariosis
Na₂EDTA	*Pseudoplatystoma reticulatum × P. corruscans*	Hemolysis and erythrocytes osmotic fragility increased in high concentration
Na₂EDTA	*Cyprinus carpio*	Hemolysis, erythrocyte deformation, membrane rupture, cell degeneration, increased hematocrit
Na₂EDTA	*Colossoma macropomum*	Hemolysis, increased erythrocyte fragility and MCH increased
Heparin	Five teleosts species	Hemolysis, when used in high concentrations, and coagulation, at low concentrations
Sodium heparin	*Pseudoplatystoma reticulatum × P. corruscans*	Coagulation after 10 hours of storage
Sodium polyanethole sulfonate	*Morone chrysops × M. saxatilis*	Agglutination of white cells and cell disruption
Sodium citrate	*Cyprinus carpio*	Increased osmotic fragility of erythrocytes

The most commonly used anticoagulants for hematological procedures in fish are heparin, EDTA, and, to a lesser extent, sodium citrate (Walencik and Witeska, 2007). Some of the forms of these drugs are sodium heparin, lithium heparin, disodium EDTA (Na EDTA), dipotassium EDTA (K EDTA), and tripotassium EDTA (K EDTA), which, in turn, act at different stages of the coagulation cascade (Harr *et al.*, 2005), which preserves the fluidity of the blood and makes it possible to perform the blood count.

Some of the restrictions on the use of heparin are its high cost and possible interference with the leukocyte staining characteristics when subjected to Romanowsky staining. Therefore, it must be diluted to such a concentration as not to prevent the penetration of the dye into the cells and, at the same time, preventing blood clotting.

The concentration of heparin in vials is in international units (IU), and therefore, when carrying out the dilution, care must be taken to verify how many IU are being used. It may be 5000 IU per 0.25 mL (ampoules) or 5000 IU per mL (vials). The use of diluted heparin (100 IU) is the most appropriate and does not cause changes in cell morphology and staining.

Heparin solution
Heparin (20,000 IU mL^{-1})......0.25 mL
Saline (0.65% NaCl) ....50.0 mL
Store in refrigerator.
Or
Heparin (5000 IU mL^{-1}) .... 1.0 mL
Saline
(0.65% NaCl) .... 50.0 mL
Store in refrigerator.

EDTA chelates factor IV (Ca^{2+}) in the coagulation cascade, being essential in various steps of coagulation and acting as a mediator as well in cell-to-cell relations during coagulation reactions (Harr *et al.*, 2005). In addition, EDTA has the advantage that it does not cause leukocyte deformation when used in blood collection. It is used as a 10% solution in distilled water.

EDTA solution (ethylenediaminetetraacetic acid)
Na EDTA..................... 3.0g
Distilled water .... 100.0 mL

Store in refrigerator.

Circulatory System of Fish

The circulatory system, responsible for blood circulation throughout the animal's body, is composed of the blood vessels (arteries, veins, and capillaries) and the heart, which is responsible for pumping this blood.

The fish heart is located in the pericardial cavity and has four compartments: (1) venous sinus, which is a thin, small, recognized discrete heart cavity; (2) auricle or atrium, with thin wall, endothelial lining, with phagocytic activity, being part of the reticuloendothelial system – RES; (3) ventricle, which has a thick, muscular wall and is irrigated by coronary vessels; it is the heart itself; and (4) arterial bulb, with thick wall and composed of elastic tissue plus smooth muscle. It acts as a passive deposit to standardize blood pressure (Fig. 2.1). There are two valves separating the venous sinus from the atrium and two separating the ventricle from the arterial bulb.

The blood circulation of fish is simple. The ventral aorta leaves the heart, sends blood to the gills, and controls blood flow. From the gills, blood is sent to the head by the carotid arteries and to the rest of the body via the dorsal aorta. After running through the whole body distributing its components, the blood is again collected from all the organs and sent back to the heart (Fig. 2.2).

Puncture of Blood Vessels or Heart

Among the different accesses for collecting blood from fish, the blood vessels located in the caudal region have been the most exploited (Fig. 2.3). Accessing the caudal blood vessel provides a quick way of obtaining a blood sample, but it is necessary to locate the vessel correctly so that it is properly cannulated, without causing many lesions in the animal. The vertebral column facilitates the use of this access, as the caudal artery and vein are located on its ventral side.

The insertion of the needle, usually inclined around 45°, is performed towards the

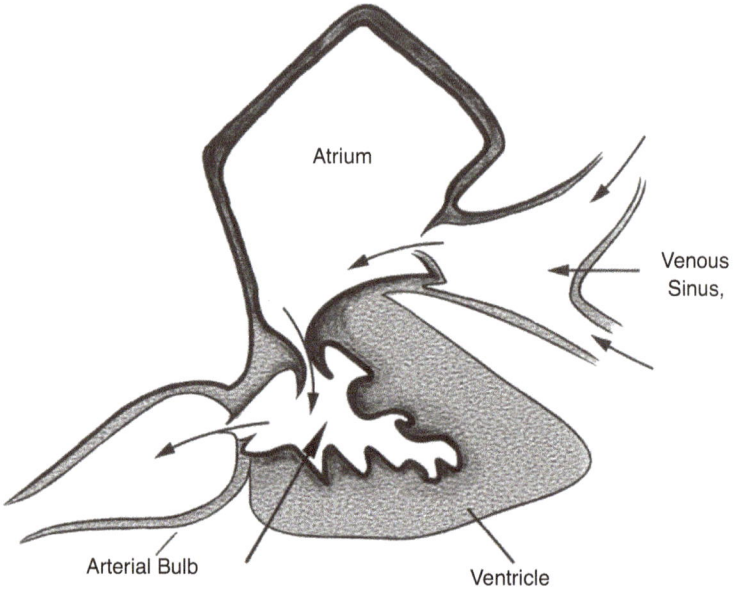

Fig. 2.1. Scheme of the heart of the catfish *Pimelodus maculatus*. Arrows – direction of blood circulation, and in the wall of the ventricle, shows the site of needle insertion for cardiac puncture. (Figure author's own.)

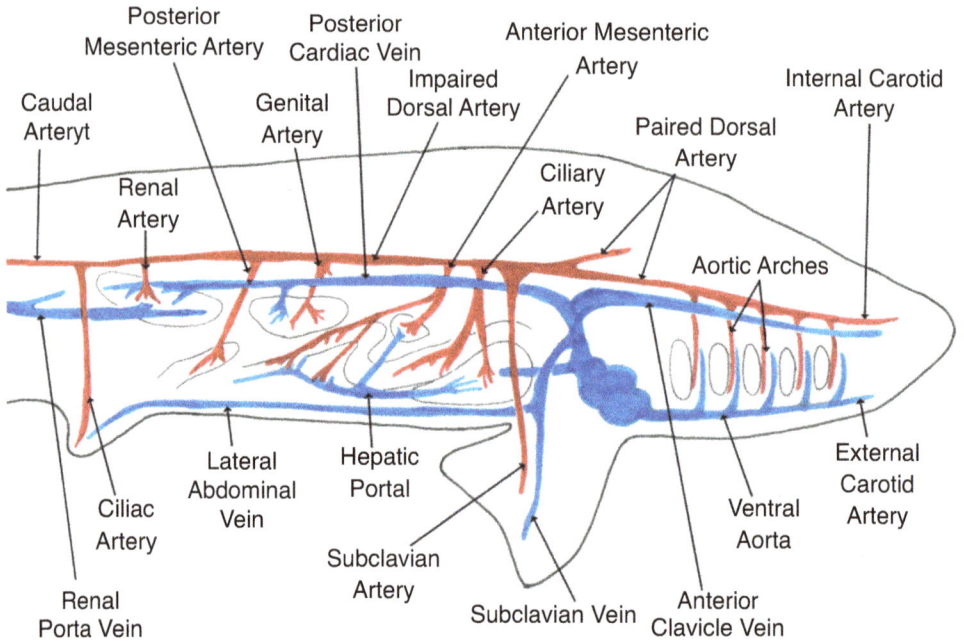

Fig. 2.2. Scheme of circulation of fish. Arterial system in red, and venous system in blue. (Figure author's own.)

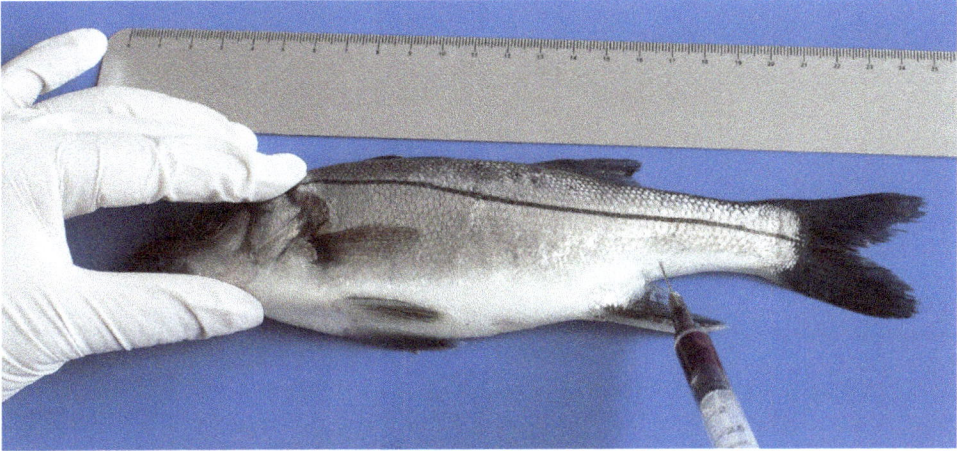

Fig. 2.3. Puncture in the caudal region in the sea bass *Centropomus parallelus* previously anesthetized with benzocaine (50 mg L–1). (Figure author's own.)

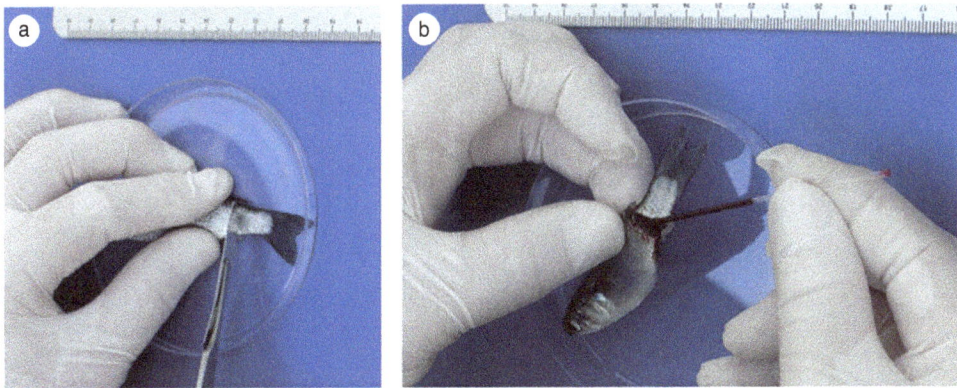

Fig. 2.4. Blood collection in lambari (*Astyanax altiparanae*) by cutting the caudal peduncle after surgical anesthesia with benzocaine (100 mg L–1). (Figure author's own.)

ventral region of the vertebral column, where the caudal artery and vein are located. The most appropriate inclination to perform this technique may vary according to the species, where it can be up to 90°, in relation to the medial line of the ventral region. The most suitable way to access blood vessels should be as comfortable as possible to the operator, since each individual can develop variations in the technique, which, in the end, will result in a quick and efficient collection.

Unnecessary negative pressure on the syringe plunger should be avoided, which could cause the rupture of red blood cells, showing up as discrete hemolysis on sedimentation of the blood cells, in addition to promoting the closure (collapse) of the cannulated vessel.

This technique may not be suitable for small ornamental fish and fingerlings in general. In these situations, anesthetic induction up to the surgical plane of the animal and the rapid and complete cut of the caudal peduncle with a scalpel are recommended (Fig. 2.4a). The blood is collected in a hematocrit capillary tube (Fig. 2.4b), and blood smears are quickly made. With the first drop of blood flowing after the cut, blood

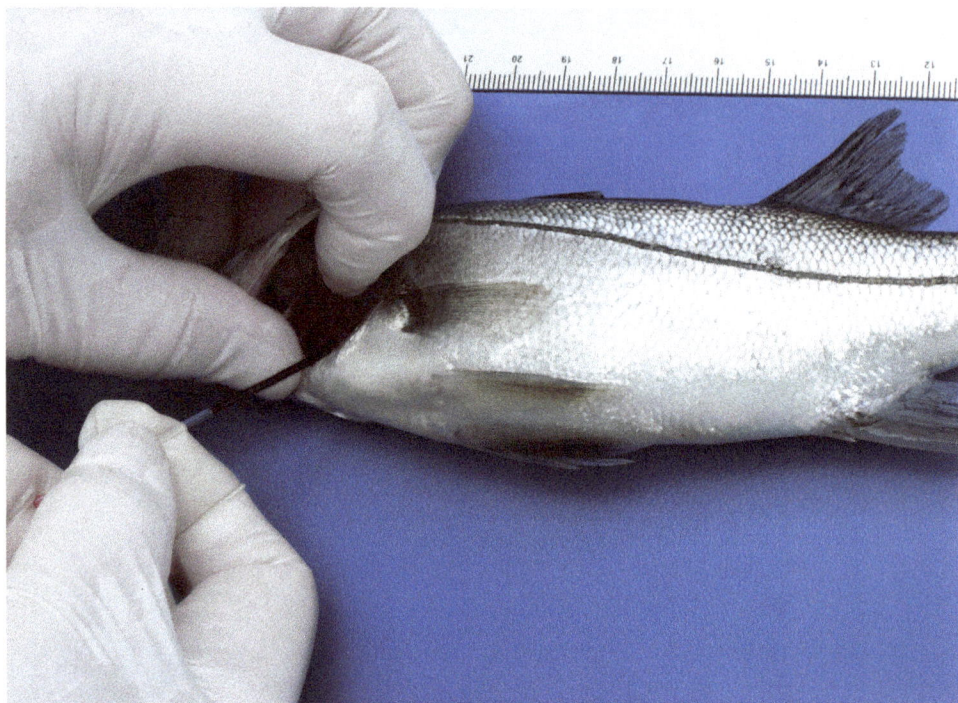

Fig. 2.5. Puncture with a hematocrit capillary tube in the catfish *Centropomus parallelus,* after surgical anesthesia with benzocaine (100 mg L–1). (Figure author's own.)

pipetting can be performed for the red blood cell count, which is essential for the white blood cell and thrombocyte counts, performed by indirect methods in fish. The main drawback of this technique is the death of the fish, in addition to contamination of the blood with extracellular fluids from nearby tissues that have been cut.

It is also possible to collect blood with the aid of a hematocrit capillary tube by puncturing a vessel at the base of the gills (Fig. 2.5). In this case, the capillary tube must be heated at one of its tips and stretched so that it has a fine tip to pierce the membrane of the gill base.

Among the accesses, gill puncture and intracardiac puncture (Fig. 2.6) are also used, especially in situations where caudal puncture cannot be performed or the anatomical peculiarities of the fish do not allow the use of this technique and make it difficult.

In stingrays, to apply this technique, the animal is placed in dorsal decubitus for appropriate containment; the needle is inserted at 90° to the fish's body in the medial region, caudal to

the gills where the heart is located (Fig. 2.7). It is important to take precautions during the handling of these fish due to the presence of stings located at the base of the tail, which are covered by venom-secreting glandular epithelium, which are used for defense (Haddad Jr. *et al.*, 2004).

To make access in blood collection of intracardiac puncture, the use of anesthetics is essential, aiming to reduce animal suffering. The collection of blood via the heart, because it is a vital organ, can lead to death of the fish when performed incorrectly, since it can produce areas of degeneration and necrosis in the myocardium.

Sometimes blood collection is not possible by the ways described above. Ranzani-Paiva *et al.* (1995b) reported that for the mullet, *Mugil platanus*, cardiac puncture was required by exposing the gills, as shown in Fig. 2.8 with *Prochilodus lineatus*, where the needle is simply inserted into the gill base and the heart with slight pressure. Blood should be drawn gently so that hemolysis does not occur.

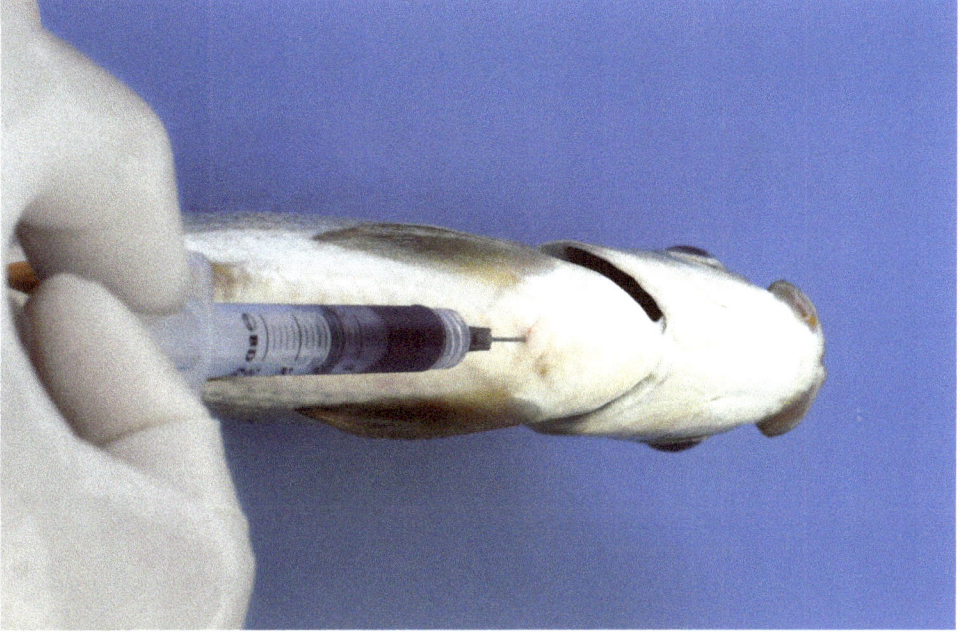

Fig. 2.6. Intracardiac puncture in juvenile of curimbatá, *Prochilodus lineatus*, previously anesthetized with benzocaine (100 mg L−1). (Figure author's own.)

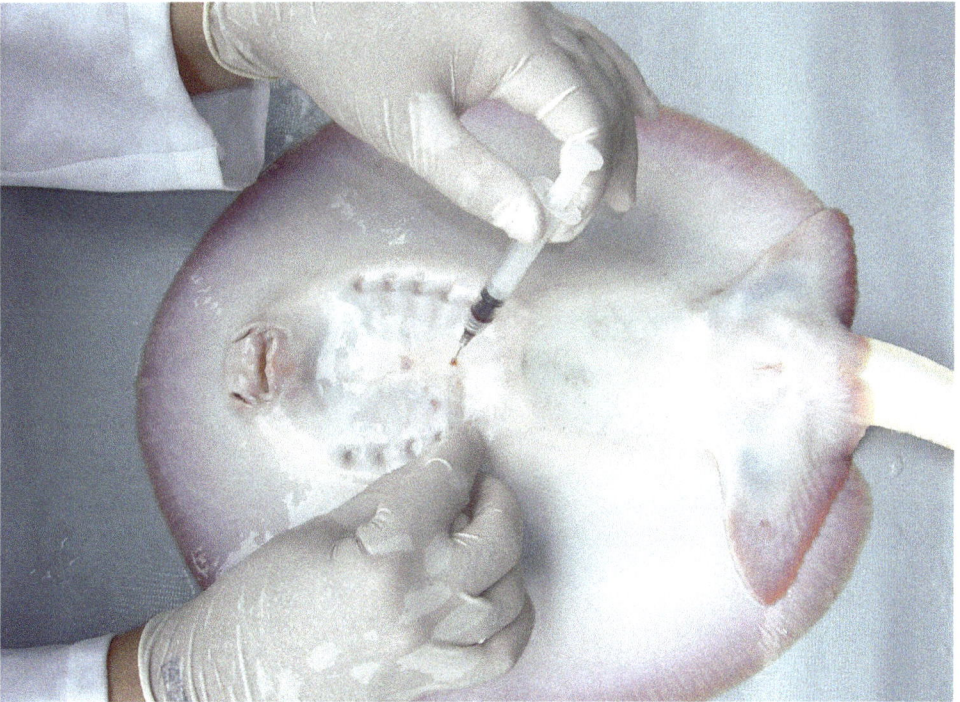

Fig. 2.7. Intracardiac puncture in a manta ray. (Photograph: Duncan, W.P.)

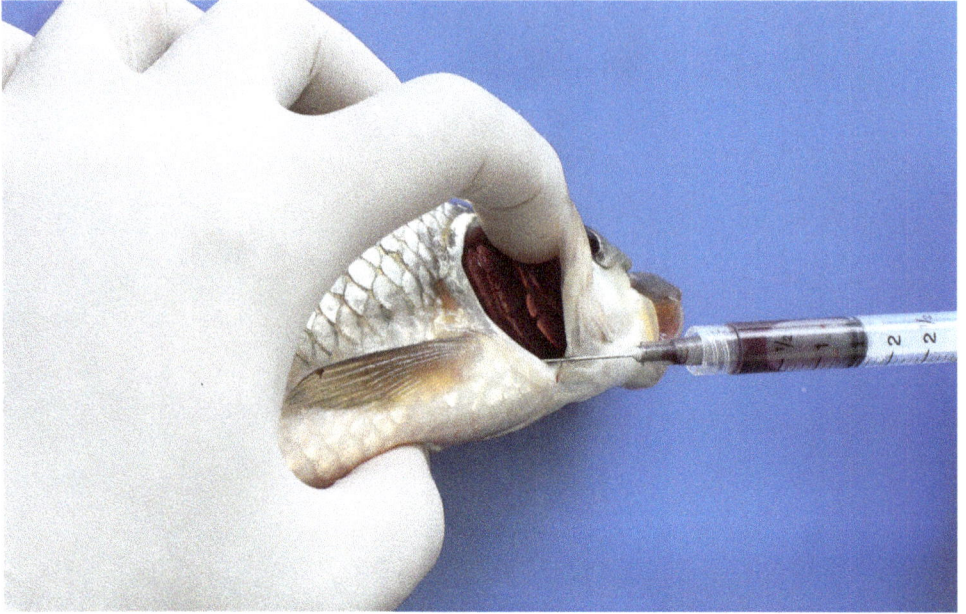

Fig. 2.8. Blood collection by cardiac puncture, via the gills of curimbatá (*Prochilodus lineatus*). (Figure author's own.)

Storage of Blood After Collection

After the blood drawing procedure using a syringe, the blood is mixed by inversion and placed in suitable tubes, generally polypropylene Eppendorf microtubes. For transfer of the blood contained in the syringe, the needle is removed and the tip of the syringe placed near the inner wall of a test tube or Eppendorf tube; slight pressure is placed on the plunger so that the blood is transferred without causing swirling, allowing it to run down the tube wall (Fig. 2.9). A widely used procedure is to leave the blood in the syringe, using it as the test tube. The plunger can be removed and the end where the needle attaches is stoppered, or the very tip of the syringe is used without removing the plunger.

The amount of blood to be collected will depend on the number of tests to be performed. For the determination of the blood count (RBC count and WBC count), 0.3 mL of blood is sufficient. When other analyses are to be performed, such as the biochemical study of plasma or serum, more blood is needed.

As there are differences due to gender, stage of gonadal maturation, age, length, and weight, among others and between individuals, the use of pools[1] is not recommended for blood tests. However, in some cases, the use of pools is necessary, in small fish, for example, in which biochemical tests are to be carried out in addition to the blood count analysis.

Procedure

1. Stress the fish as little as possible, so remove it from the stabilization containers and handle it gently to prevent it from thrashing about.
2. The material used should be clean, well sterilized, and preferably disposable.
3. The choice of site to draw blood is up to the ability and experience of the operator.
4. The vessel should be punctured immediately to avoid moving the needle in the animal.
5. Blood should flow easily without exerting too much pressure on the syringe plunger.
6. Mix blood slowly and gently to avoid cell lysis.

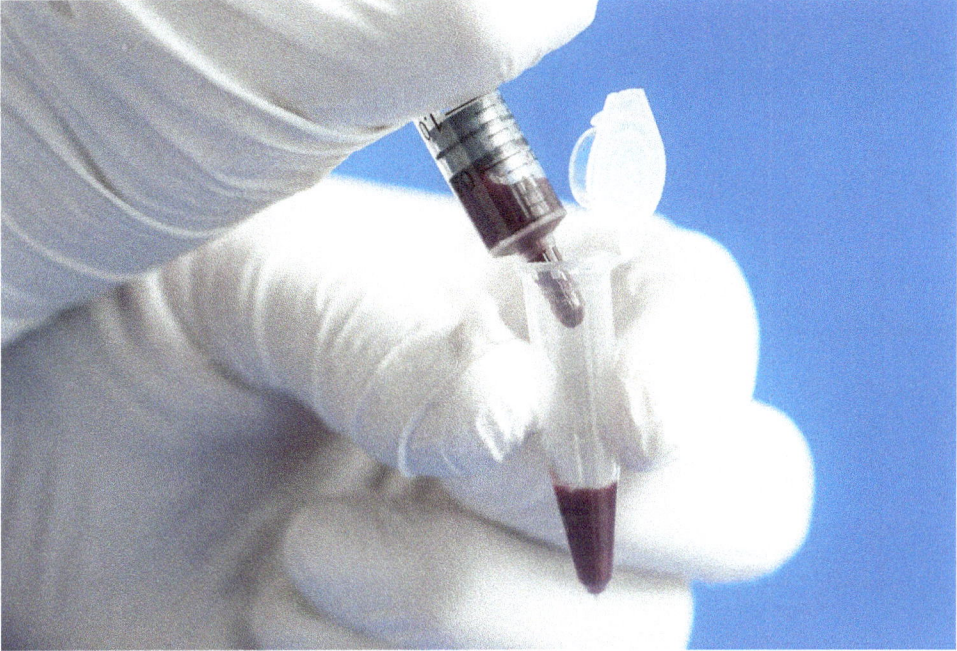

Fig. 2.9. Placing blood in a polypropylene microtube. (Figure author's own.)

7. Blood smears must be made immediately after drawing blood before clotting.

Lysis of the blood cells occurs by mechanical action or when they are placed in a hypotonic solution and enlarge until rupture of the cell wall. The reverse is called crenation, when the cells are placed in a hypertonic solution and lose liquid to the medium. This care for material collection is very important because the quality of the results depends on the quality of the blood collection. It is recommended that blood smears be made soon after blood collection, as detailed in Chapter IV.

The method to be used should be chosen and practiced before beginning the study or the examination to be done. Once chosen, it should always be the same, so that there is standardization and uniformity in the results.

Note

[1] When working with small animals, such as ornamental fish, tadpoles or fry of various species, a sufficient amount of material from a single animal is often not obtained, so it is necessary to collect blood from more than one animal, mixing the samples in the same container and then treating it as a pool.

3 Hemogram

Part 1: Erythrogram

The complete blood count (CBC) is a set of tests that are performed to determine the number of different cells in the blood, the volume of red blood cells (RBCs) occupy, and the amount of hemoglobin inside them. The CBC is divided into three parts: RBC count, white blood cells (WBC) count, and thrombocyte count.

The RBC count consists of the following tests: RBC number; hematocrit and hemoglobin concentration; and calculation of RBC indices, mean corpuscular volume (MCV), mean corpuscular hemoglobin (MCH), and mean corpuscular hemoglobin concentration (MCHC). The WBC count consists of the relative and absolute numbers of the different leukocytes, and the thrombocyte count consists of the number of thrombocytes.

When the blood cells settle, three layers form. The upper, liquid phase is represented by serum or plasma; the middle is white, composed of WBCs plus thrombocytes; and the lower one is red, composed of RBCs, which represent approximately 45% of the total blood volume (Fig. 3.1).

The blood is composed of a liquid medium, the plasma, containing the three classes of blood cells: RBCs (or erythrocytes), WBCs (lymphocytes, monocytes, neutrophils, basophils, eosinophils, and special granulocyte cells [SGC, PAS-GL]), and thrombocytes (similar to mammalian platelets).

The liquid phase is amorphous and termed plasma or serum. Plasma is the blood without cells, obtained by centrifugation when an anticoagulant is used. Serum is blood without cells and with little or no substances used in coagulation (such as fibrinogen that forms a fibrin network that holds the cells and thrombocytes in its mesh – the clot) and is obtained when blood is collected without the use of an anticoagulant.

Plasma is composed of 90% water, 7% proteins (globulins and albumin), and various solutes (electrolytes, such as carbonate, sodium, potassium, calcium, and phosphate), metabolites, hormones, enzymes, and so on.

Red Blood Cell Counting (RBC)

Erythrocytes are the most abundant cells in the circulation; their main function is the transport of oxygen and carbon dioxide through the binding of O_2 to hemoglobin, forming oxyhemoglobin in the respiratory organs, followed by the exchange of O_2 for tissue CO_2 (Ranzani-Paiva, 2007)

For RBCs to be counted, it is necessary to dilute the blood due to their high number. Special solutions are used for this purpose that do not alter the shape or volume of the cells, and dilution is carried out using special pipettes: the Thoma pipette (Figs 3.2 and 3.3) or an automatic pipette (Fig. 3.4).

The Thoma pipette consists of a graduated capillary tube with a bulb dilated 100 times more than that of the capillary (in the case of RBC pipettes) at the top. Inside this bulb is a small glass bead (white or red), which facilitates mixing of the suspension and whose volume is not counted in the bulb volume. The white or red color of the bead indicates the type of dilution: white for smaller dilution (1:20) used in WBC counts, which are very much lower in number; red for greater dilution (1:200) indicated for RBC counts. A flexible rubber tube is attached to the tapered top of both pipettes to allow aspiration of the blood and the diluent liquid. This technique requires great skill from the technician

Methods for Haematological Analysis in Fish (Maria José Ranzani Paiva *et al.*)
DOI: 10.1079/9781836991762.0003

Plasma or Serum ⟶

White Blood Cells
and Thrombocytes ⟶

Red Blood Cells ⟶

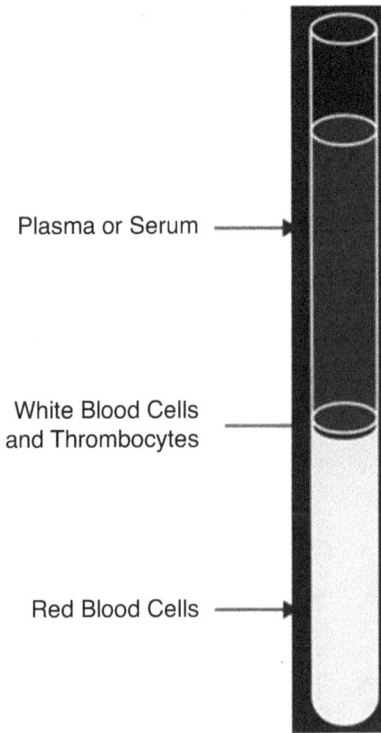

Fig. 3.1. Blood layers after centrifugation or sedimentation of blood cells. (Figure author's own.)

and is susceptible to significant errors. The blood cannot exceed the 0.5 mark, because the cells adhere to the wall of the capillary, nor the diluent of the 101 marks.

In mammals, the leukocyte count is also performed using a hemocytometer or in a Neubauer chamber, with the aid of a Thoma pipette for WBC counts. For fish, this technique is not recommended because of the erythrocyte nucleus. In the dilution for total counting of WBCs in mammals, a solution is used that lyses the cells, leaving only the nuclei of the leukocytes. In fish, if this solution were used, the nuclei of all cells would remain, which makes counting impossible.

For automatic pipettes, dilution is simpler. Care must be taken to follow the manufacturer's instructions for a perfect dilution (Annex 1). Whenever necessary, request assistance to

improve the technique. These pipettes require constant cleaning and calibration.

The determination of the number of erythrocytes, widely used in hematological surveys of mammals, is not often done without errors in fish, due to the presence of both leukocytes and nucleated erythrocytes. The diluents commonly used in the total WBC count in mammals lyse the cells, leaving only the WBC nuclei to be counted, since the erythrocytes are anucleated, as stated above. To obtain the total number of erythrocytes, the number of leukocytes is subtracted from the total cell count in the hemocytometer (Neubauer chamber).

The most widely used method for counting RBCs is the visual method, performed in a Neubauer chamber (Fig. 3.5). This chamber consists of a thick glass rectangular slide, containing two reticles in the central portion separated longitudinally by a deep groove on the slide. Transversally, four grooves separate three platforms: central, where the grids are, there is a depression of 0.1 mm in relation to the sides, giving depth to the chamber, bordered on top by a coverslip especially adapted to firmly sit on the lateral platforms (Fig. 3.6).

The grid in the improved Neubauer chamber (Figs 3.7 and 3.8) is a $3 \times 3\,mm^2$, divided into nine areas of $1\,mm^2$, where four lateral are divided into 20 squares each, and the central square is divided into 25 squares of $1/25\,mm^2$, each subdivided into 16 small squares of $1/400\,mm^2$ totaling 400 tiny squares of $0.1\,mm^3$ in the central area.

The blood is diluted 1:200 using both the Thoma pipette and the automatic pipette. Both of them are used with manual counting. Another technique is to perform the counting with a computerized image, where a specific software is used for this purpose. In addition to these methods, automated devices widely employed in mammalian clinical hematology are sometimes adapted by researchers for use in fish but with questionable results.

To dilute with automatic pipettes, 2 mL of diluent (Hayem's solution, 0.65% NaCl, or formaldehyde-citrate solution) is used (Fig. 3.9). The blood, stored in polypropylene tubes, is gently mixed, then the reverse blood pipetting is performed (see Annex I). Clean the blood from

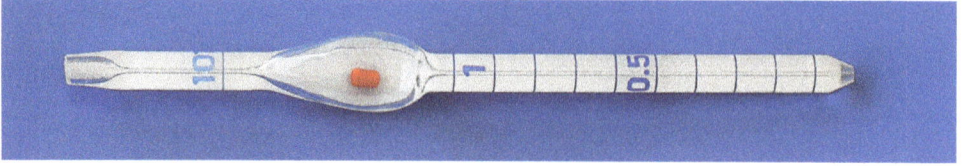

Fig. 3.2. Thoma pipette for blood dilution used in RBC counting. (Figure author's own.)

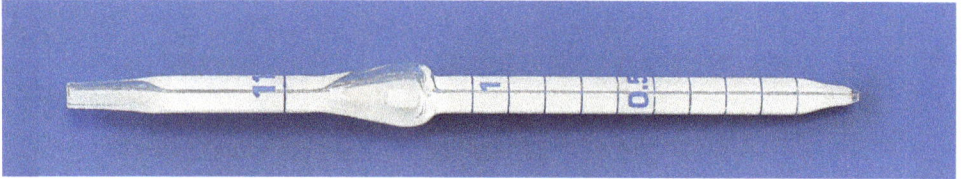

Fig. 3.3. Thoma pipet for blood dilution used in WBC counting. (Figure author's own.)

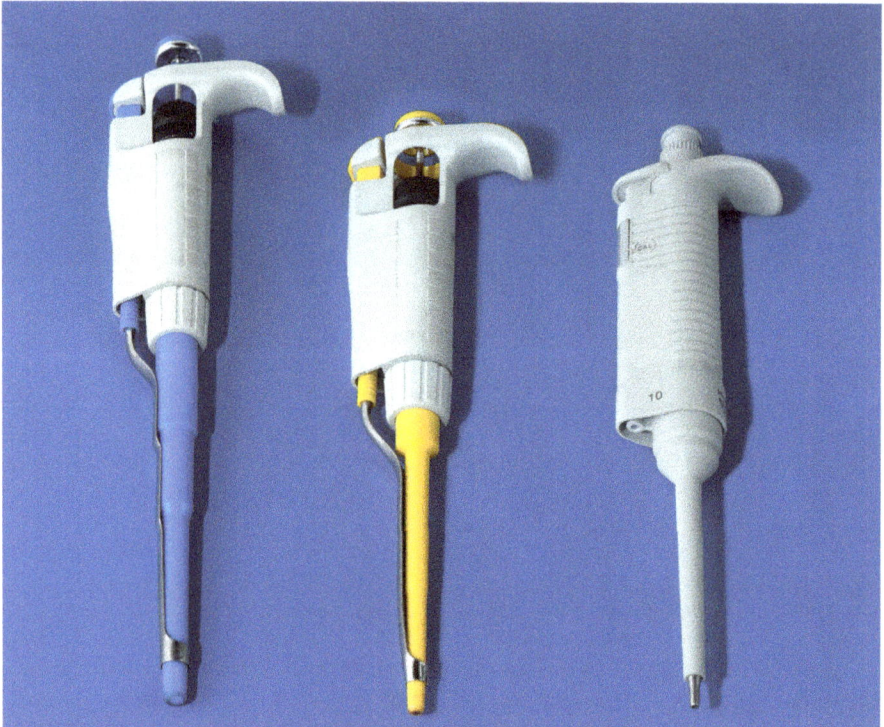

Fig. 3.4. Automatic pipettes of various volumes for blood dilution. (Figure author's own.)

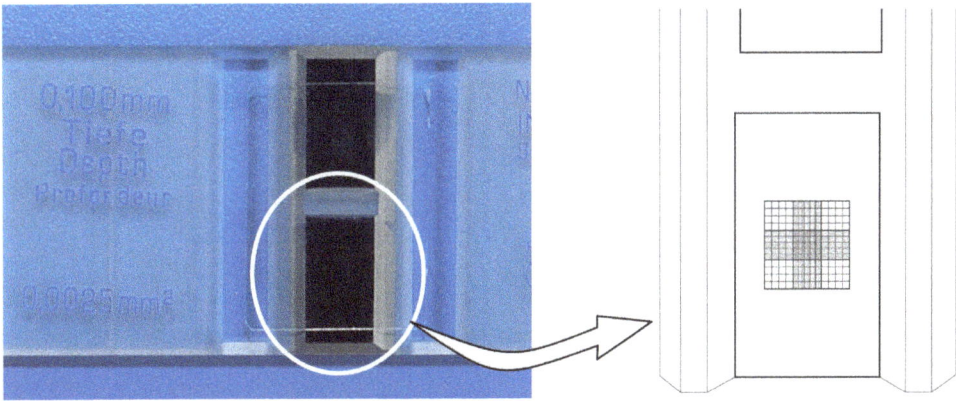

Fig. 3.5. Neubauer chamber and coverslip, for counting total cells, in detailed scheme of grid on each side of the slide. (Figure author's own.)

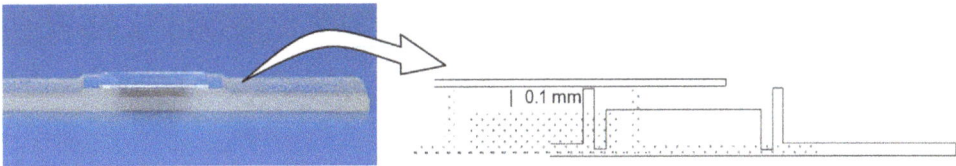

Fig. 3.6. Profile of Neubauer chamber, coverslip, in detailed scheme of side view. (Figure author's own.)

the tip with gauze or tissue, taking care not to touch the tip of the paper, as blood loss may occur. After pipetting, the blood suspension plus the hemodiluent is homogenized immediately, especially when using formaldehyde-citrate, as clumping of cells may occur, which compromises the red cell count. It should be noted that it is important to do this procedure in duplicate by diluting the blood of the same animal in two pipettes and separate tubes.

Hayem's solution
Mercuric chloride 0.5g
Sodium sulfate 5.0g
Sodium chloride 1.0g
Distilled water .... 200.0 mL
Store in refrigerator.

Saline or physiological solution (0.65% NaCl)
Sodium chloride 0.65g
Distilled water .... 100.00 mL

Formal-citrate

Formaldehyde (37%) .... 3.0 mL
Sodium citrate 2.9g
Distilled water .... 100.0 mL

Hayem's solution
Mercuric chloride 0.5g
Sodium sulfate 5.0g
Sodium chloride 1.0g
Distilled water .... 200.0 mL
Store in refrigerator.

Saline or physiological solution (0.65% NaCl)
Sodium chloride 0.65g
Distilled water .... 100.00 mL

Formol-citrate
Formaldehyde (37%) .... 3.0 mL
Sodium citrate 2.9g
Distilled water .... 100.0 mL

Procedure for counting

1. Mix the tubes gently, allowing some swirling for a few seconds to resuspend RBCs evenly,

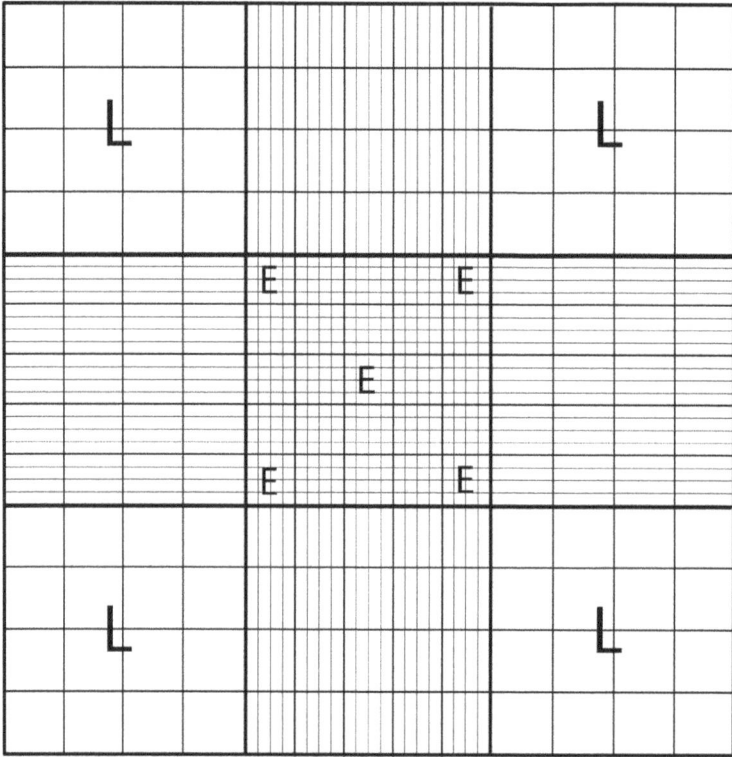

Fig. 3.7. Grid of Neubauer chamber for counting erythrocytes (E) and leukocytes (L). (Figure author's own.)

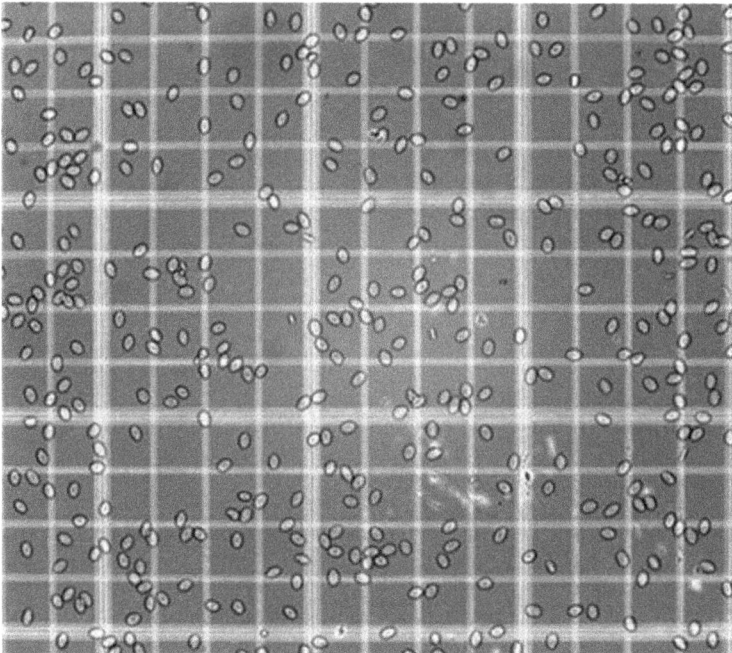

Fig. 3.8. Neubauer chamber grid with diluted blood. (Figure author's own.)

then fill the chamber. If there is a problem with the filling, clean the chamber, mix the tube again for a few seconds, and fill it one more time.

2. Initially, the coverslip is placed on the platforms of the chamber, with slight pressing for good adherence. Some technicians moisten the platforms with a little saliva to secure the coverslip.

3. This procedure is unnecessary and can alter the distance between the chamber and the coverslip.

4. Fill each chamber grid with diluted blood.

5. The chamber filling is good when there is no excess or insufficient liquid and there are no air bubbles.

6. Let the slide stand in a humid container for a few seconds to allow the cells to settle.

7. Place the chamber slide on the microscope. View under low power to see if cells are evenly distributed, and count cells in five small squares of the grid (Fig. 3.10). A $10\times$ or $40\times$ objective and $10\times$ eyepiece are used for counting. In any grid, cells lying on one side are counted and those on the opposite side are not (Fig. 3.11).

8. Count two grids and take the average. The result is expressed as cells $\mu L-1$.

9. Do not delay counting, as this may cause the liquid in the chamber to dry. If more time is needed, it is recommended that moist container be used for storage (Fig. 3.12). A slide that has become partially dry should not be used.

10. The difference between the two counts should not be over 25%; otherwise, new dilutions need to be done.

If all the RBCs present in the central square of the Neubauer chamber (divided into 400 cells) were counted, the exact number of RBCs in 0.01 mm3 would be obtained, since the height of this chamber is 0.1 mm. To determine the number of cells per mm3, the value obtained would need to be multiplied by 10. Multiplying this value obtained by the dilution gives the absolute count. However, since only five squares are counted, it is necessary to calculate the final number of RBCs.

It is calculated as follows:

Number of RBCs = number of cells counted ×dilution (200) × height coverslip (10) × 5 (which is the number of squares counted).

This simplifies as follows:

Number of RBCs = number of cells counted × 10,000

In practice, the number of cells counted is multiplied by 10^4 or 10^6.

For example: 250 cells are counted in the chamber, so the final number of RBCs is 250×104 mm^{-3} of blood = $2,500,000$ cells μL^{-1} of blood. This value can be expressed as

$$2.50 \times 104\,\mu L^{-1} \text{ or } 2.50 \times 106\,\mu L^{-1}.$$

When using mirrored Neubauer chambers, avoid rubbing them during drying with a cloth or paper. It is recommended that the chambers be dried only by contact and light pressure with an absorbent surface. This is important because with the friction of the mirrored glass, an electric field is created, which prevents or greatly hinders the proper filling of the grid.

Table 3.1.

Causes of error
• Blood not well mixed;
• Clotted blood, with partial coagulation;
• Not careful to remove excess blood from tip;
• Amount of blood used is too small, with large dilution by anticoagulant;
• Field errors – irregular distribution of cells in grid;
• Pipetting error – minimized by use of automatic pipettes;
• Lack of technician experience and care during the procedure.

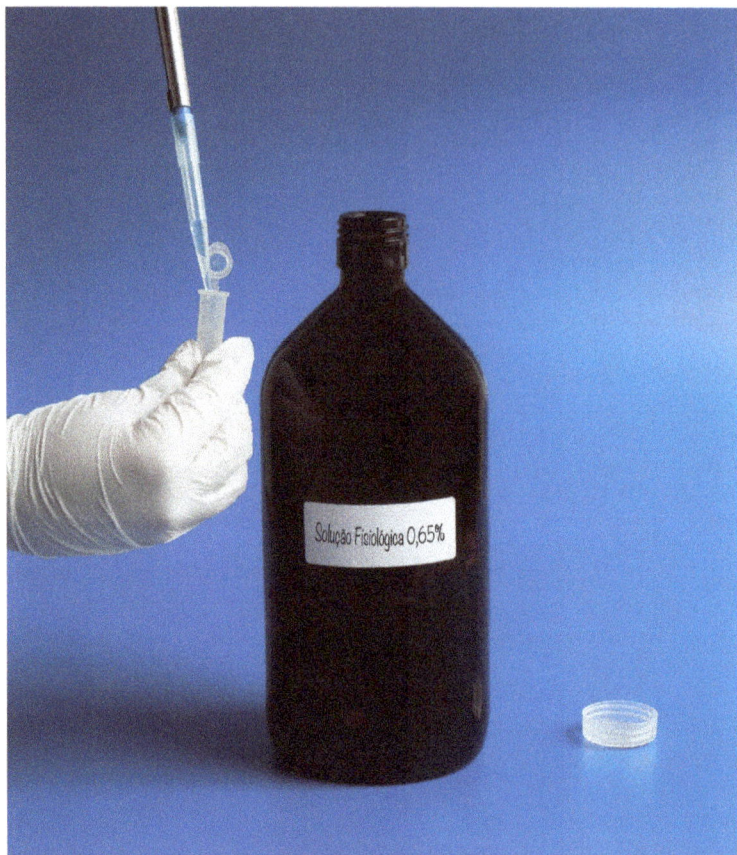

Fig. 3.9. Dilution for counting RBCs. Hayem's, 0.65% NaCl or formol-citrate solution. (Figure author's own.)

Hematocrit

The hematocrit percentage reflects the proportion of RBCs in the blood relative to the amount of leukocytes, thrombocytes, and blood plasma. It is characterized by being one of the most reliable hematological parameters due to the low variability and low margin of errors during its determination. In addition, the microhematocrit technique, validated by Goldenfarb *et al.* (1971), is widely used. To determine this parameter, the blood must be well mixed.

Procedure

1. The heparinized microcapillary tube is filled with two-thirds of its total volume (Fig. 3.13a)

and sealed at one end (Fig. 3.13b). Sealing can be done with modeling clay, a Bunsen burner flame, or in some similar way. With the burner, one must be very careful when using fire in the laboratory environment and avoid warming the blood in the tube, which could cause hemolysis and increase the MCV. Accordingly, this sealing method is little used and rarely recommended.

2. After sealing, the microcapillary tube is placed in a hematocrit microcentrifuge, and the sealed end is set against the rubber ring lining the plate (Fig 3.14), thereby preventing the loss of samples due to breakage of the microcapillary tube during centrifugation.

3. The tubes are centrifuged at 12,000 rpm for 5 min. The time of centrifugation should be

Table 3.2.

Causes of error

- Blood not well mixed.
- Partial clotting of blood.
- Small amount of blood and large dilution by anticoagulant.
- Formation of gelatinous mass.
- Lack of experience and care on the part of the technician during the process.
- Incorrect calculation of correction factor.

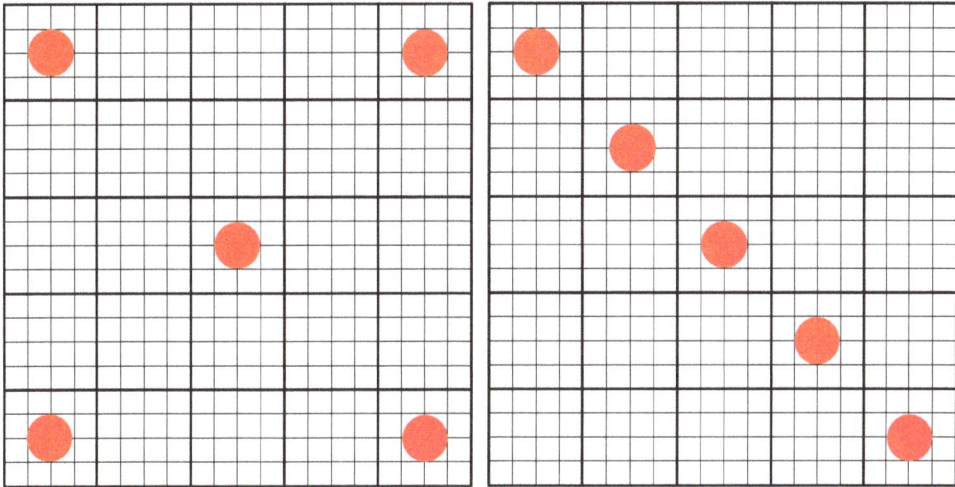

Fig. 3.10. Scheme for counting RBCs in Neubauer chamber. Choose one of two schemes. (Figure author's own.)

previously determined by comparing different times, until results are stable, with the three layers visible (Fig. 3.15).

4. For reading the tube, align the meniscus of the plasma with the line that represents 100% on the chart and the top of the RBCs with the line that represents 0% on the chart. The height of the RBC column on the table corresponds to hematocrit percentage (Fig. 3.16).

5. The result is expressed in percentage of RBCs in relation to total blood.

The centrifugation time should be tested when starting the study of a new species. After a certain time of centrifugation, the compacted cells are measured and the same capillary tube is centrifuged again for a longer time and re-read. If both readings are the same, the shortest time is what should be used. If the reading is higher,

new centrifugations need to be done until the measurement stabilizes. The microhematocrit is also a method used in the detection of flagellated protozoan parasites in the blood, when the parasitosis is at low intensity. The parasites are concentrated in the leukocyte layer, and the capillary tubes can be directly observed under a regular light microscope, at low magnification ($20\times$ or $40\times$). The parasites are easily observed due to their active movements (Eiras et al., 2000).

After measurement of the hematocrit, a biochemical parameter can be determined from the plasma remaining in the microcapillary after centrifugation. This parameter is the total plasma protein (TPP) content, which can be measured by refractometry. For this procedure, the microcapillary must be broken above the leukocyte layer and the plasma placed on the prism

Table 3.3.

Causes of error
• Blood not well mixed.
• Partial clotting.
• Small amount of blood used, with large dilution of blood by anticoagulant.
• Warming of the microtube when using a flame for sealing.
• Delay in reading, where cells spread or swell and retract due to cell respiration.
• Error in reading the chart, including the buffy coat with RBCs.
• Lack of experience and care of the technician during the procedure.

of the refractometer. At each analysis, the prism of the refractometer is washed with distilled water and calibrated at the point corresponding to 0g dL^{-1} of the TPP scale.

Hemoglobin Concentration

Determination of the hemoglobin level is one of the simplest and most common ways to determine the occurrence of anemia. The methods used are those of acid hematin, oxyhemoglobin, and cyanmethemoglobin. The latter is the most used, although it gives abnormally high readings, due to the formation of a gelatinous mass, caused by the presence of the nuclei of fish erythrocytes. However, after centrifugation, this mass can be removed using a Pasteur pipette.

This method consists of adding whole blood to a solution containing potassium ferricyanide and potassium cyanide (Collier, 1944). Potassium ferricyanide transforms the hemoglobin iron from the ferrous (bivalent) state into the ferric (trivalent) state, forming methemoglobin, which in turn combines with potassium cyanide to produce a stable pigment, cyanmethemoglobin. The color intensity of this mixture is then determined in a spectrophotometer. The result is expressed in g dL^{-1}.

The dilution of blood for the determination of hemoglobin level is done with a micropipette or Sahli pipette (Fig. 3.17), which is connected to a rubber tube. The blood is aspirated by the technician by mouth. Currently, automatic pipettes are widely used because of their precision and greater safety in handling blood (Fig. 3.14).

Procedure

1. Mix blood for reverse pipetting of 20 μL (Annex I), wipe the blood from the tip with gauze or tissue, taking care not to touch the tip with tissue, in which some blood can be lost to the tissue.
2. Dilute blood with 5 mL of Drabkin reagent.
3. Seal the assay tube with Parafilm.
4. Mix and let stand for 15 min, at least.
5. Centrifuge at 3500 rpm for 5 min.
6. Read absorbance in a spectrophotometer at 540 nm, against the Drabkin reagent (blank).

The absorbance is read in the spectrophotometer. When reading transmittance, it must be converted to absorbance by the calculation: $2^{-\log 10}$ of the transmittance or the reading can be done directly in absorbance. The final calculation of the hemoglobin concentration is done by multiplying the absorbance obtained in the sample by the correction factor calculated from the standard curve. Every time a new solution is prepared, the correction factor should be calculated anew, which can be done with commercial kits.

Hb level = Absorbance of sample × correction factor (expressed in g dL^{-1})
For example: Hb = 0.250 × 34.86 = 8.72g dL^{-1}

Cyanmethemoglobin reagent (Drabkin):
Potassium ferricyanide .... 100.0 mg
Sodium bicarbonate......................... 2.0 mg
Potassium cyanide .... 50.00 mg
Distilled water (q.s.p.) .... 1000.00 mL

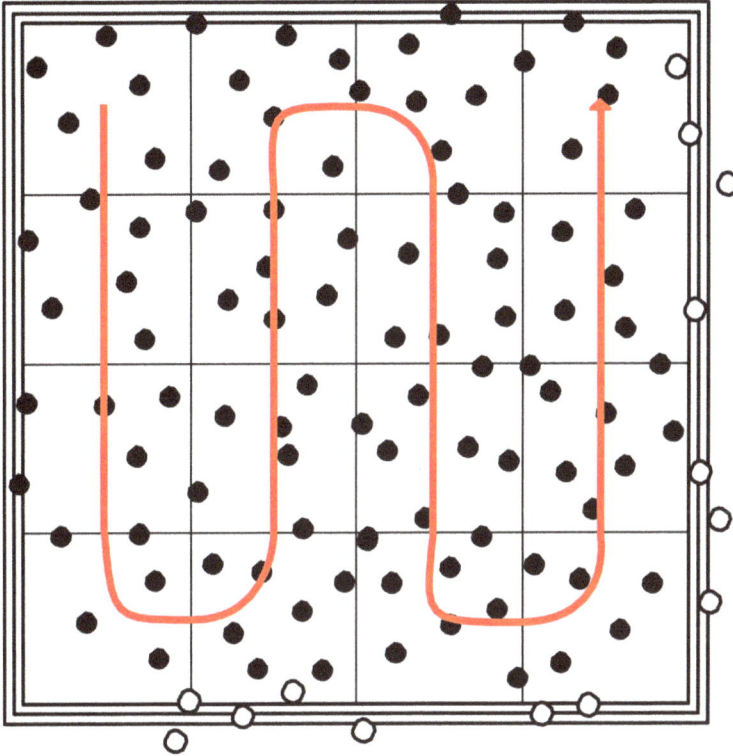

Fig. 3.11. Conventional scheme for counting RBCs in one of the small squares of the Neubauer chamber. Filled circles are cells to be counted; open circles are cells that are not counted. Arrow indicates the direction of counting (adapted from Matos and Matos, 1995.)

Stored in refrigerator in an amber bottle.

Extreme care is needed when handling this solution, as cyanide intoxication is lethal. Pipetting this solution should never be done by mouth, only with an automatic pipette. In addition, this solution should be well labeled and kept in a safe place, protected from light.

Calculation of RBC Indices

In hematology, there are three RBC indices that are of great use in the evaluation and classification of anemias in general. These indices are relations between the hematocrit and number of erythrocytes; hemoglobin level and number of erythrocytes; and hemoglobin level and hematocrit (Wintrobe, 1934).

- Mean corpuscular volume (MCV) evaluates the volume of erythrocytes.

$$MCV = \frac{Hematocrit \times 10}{Number\ of\ erythrocytes\ (\times 10^6\ \mu L^{-1})} = fL$$

- Mean corpuscular hemoglobin concentration (MCHC) is related to the concentration of hemoglobin in the erythrocytes.

$$MCV = \frac{Hematocrit \times 100}{Hematocrit} = g\ dL^{-1}$$

These indices are used for the classification of anemias, a condition in which the capacity of the blood to transport oxygen to the tissues is reduced. The lack of oxygen in organs is known as hypoxia. Anemias are characterized by a decreased number of RBCs, RBC volume (hematocrit), and hemoglobin concentration in

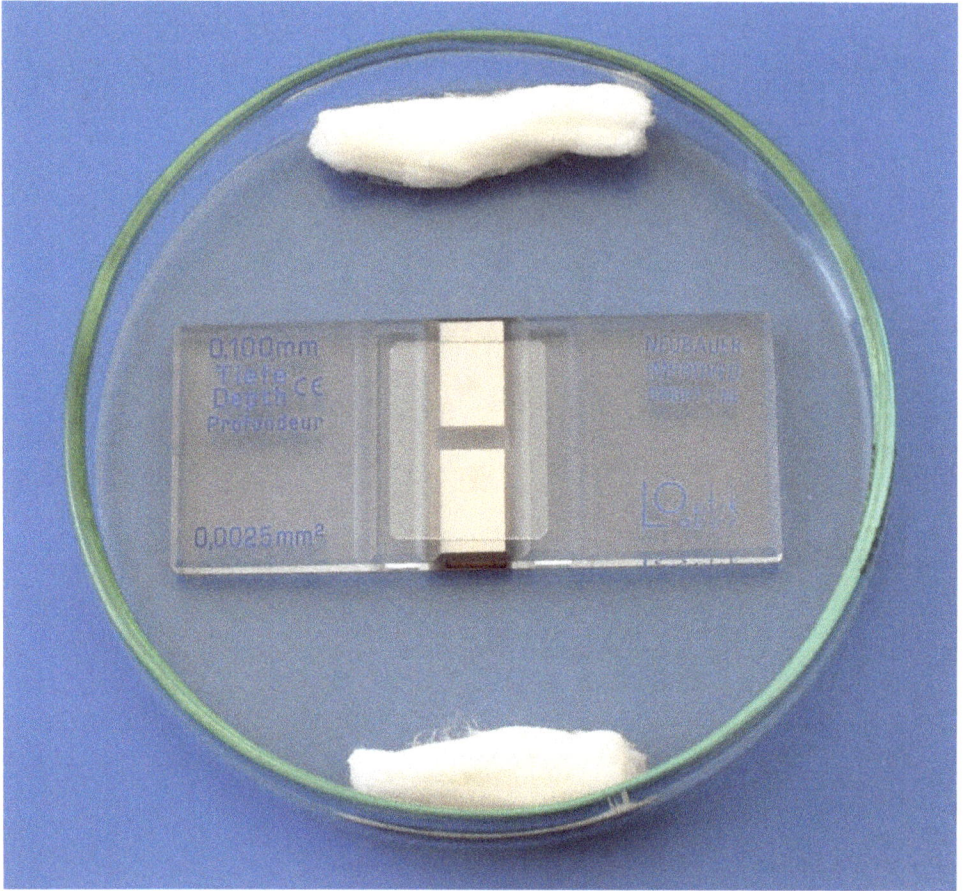

Fig. 3.12. Moist container for storing the Neubauer chamber before counting. (Figure author's own.)

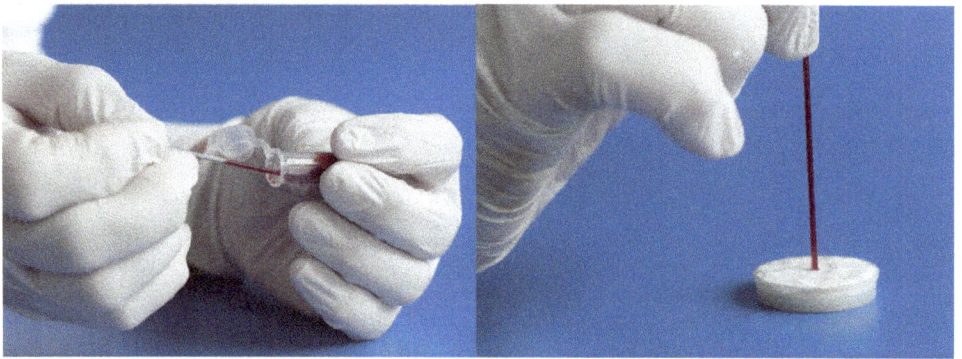

Fig. 3.13. Procedure for filling (a) and sealing (b) the microcapillary tube. (Figure author's own.)

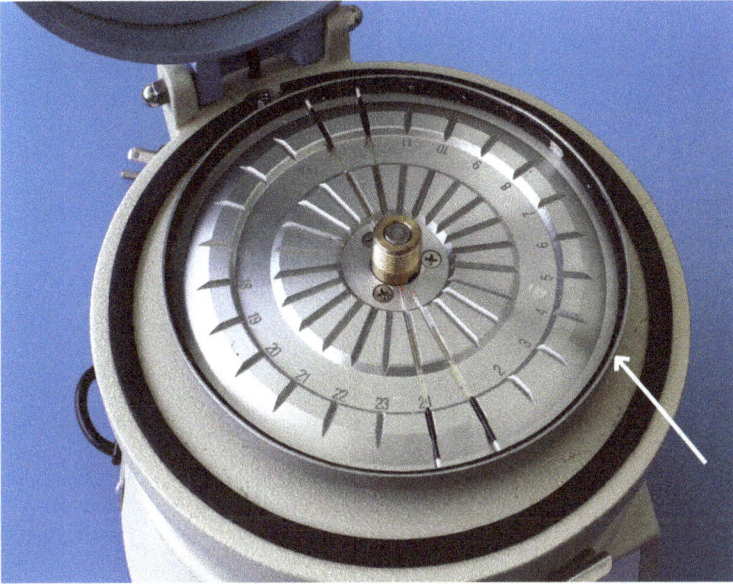

Fig. 3.14. Placing the capillary tubes in the microcentrifuge plate, where they have to be against the rubber band (arrow) to avoid loss of samples. (Figure author's own.)

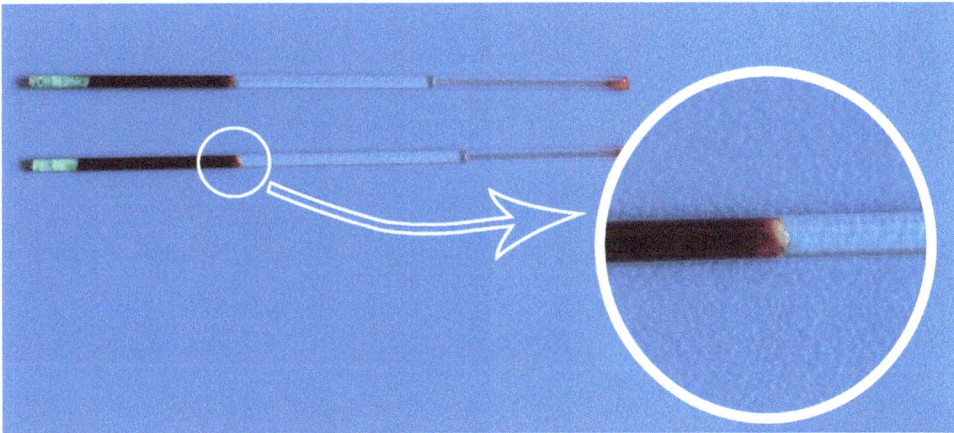

Fig. 3.15. Hematocrit capillary tube after centrifugation, visualizing the three layers of blood. (Figure author's own.)

RBCs. The number of RBCs can be normal, but each can have a low hemoglobin level.

Anemia can be caused by

- loss of blood (acute hemorrhage, aplastic anemia, iron deficiency anemia in initial phase, secondary to chronic diseases);

- reduced or defective erythropoiesis due to genetic problems, for example, erythrocyte membrane defects and enzymatic defects (glucose-6-phosphate dehydrogenase deficiency). Anemia due to selective suppression of erythrogenesis can be caused by chronic infectious disease, parasitic disease, and organic or tissue disorders;

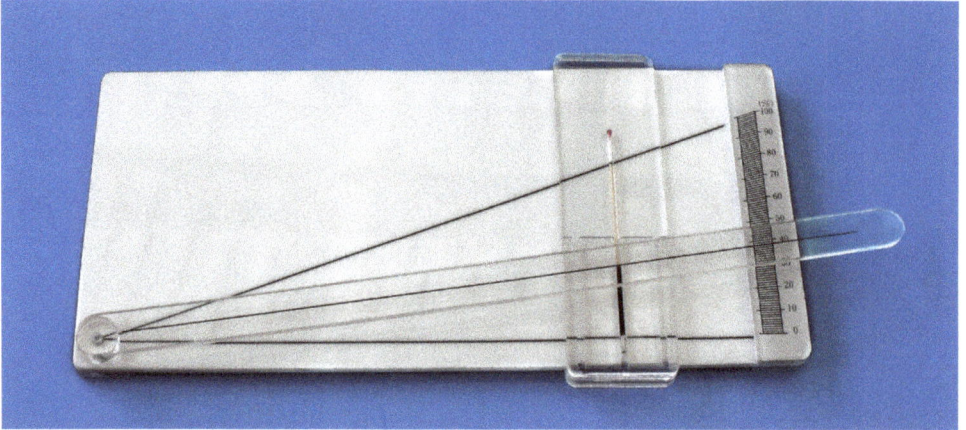

Fig. 3.16. Chart for reading hematocrit. (Figure author's own.)

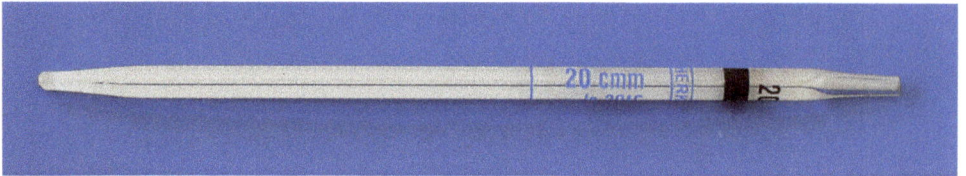

Fig. 3.17. Sahli pipette for dilution of blood in determination of hemoglobin level. (Figure author's own.)

- production of erythrocytes with insufficient hemoglobin, generally due to a deficiency of Fe (iron deficiency), Cu, Co, thiamine, vitamin B12 (pernicious anemia, vegetarian diet, tapeworms), folate, pyridoxine, and low-protein diet;
- accelerated destruction of erythrocytes by clearance.[1] Besides these parameters, the morphological analysis of the erythrocytes in blood smears is also useful for etiological diagnosis.

Classification of anemias by size of erythrocytes

Like in mammals, anemias in fish can be classified according to the size of the erythrocytes, inferred by the MCV, as follows:

- normocytic anemia: it is within the normal range of MCV. Causes: malignant tumors, chronic infectious diseases, radiation (X-rays), nephritis;
- microcytic anemia: it is generally hypochromic, due to selective suppression of erythropoiesis (iron deficiency anemia); it is below the normal range;
- macrocytic anemia: it is above the normal range and can be transitory – animal in a phase of recuperation from great loss of blood; true – interference with erythrocyte maturation, where the causes can be deficiency of vitamin B12, folic acid, and so on;
- megaloblastic anemia: it can be caused by lack of vitamin B12 and use of certain medications that inhibit the formation of erythrocytes;
- anisocytosis: many erythrocytes of abnormal sizes;
- poikilocytes: abnormally shaped erythrocytes;
- spherocytes: small size and spherical erythrocytes;

- acanthocytes: erythrocytes showing spiked cell membrane;
- polycythemia: increased number of erythrocytes, generally accompanied by increased hemoglobin and hematocrit;
- relative polycythemia: when there is hemoconcentration, that is, decrease in plasma volume, where the causes can be a reduction in intake of liquids, passage of water from plasma to interstitial spaces and shock.
- transitory polycythemia: disappears when the causal agent is eliminated, where the causes can be acute hemorrhage, reduction in O_2, exercise, emotions, and use of sympathomimetic drugs.
- absolute polycythemia: true increase in erythrocytes;
- erythrocytosis (increased number of erythrocytes) with polycythemia;
- erythremia (decreased number of erythrocytes – cause unknown).

Classification of anemias by decrease in haemoglobin amount

- normochromic: normal amounts of hemoglobin;

- hypochromic: cells show hemoglobin levels below normal;
- polychromasia: large and small erythrocytes in the same smear and with different coloration;
- anachromasia: whitish central area.

Classification of anemias according to Wintrobe

- morphological anemias: based on the classification of erythrocytes as well as MCV, MCH, and MCHC;
- etiological anemias: they can be anemias from loss of blood: acute hemorrhage due to intoxication, trauma or surgery, chronic hemorrhage caused by neoplasia with bleeding, vitamin C and K deficiency, prothrombin deficiency, gastrointestinal lesions, and internal and external parasites. Hemolytic anemia can be infectious (caused by bacteria), toxic (due to intoxication by Cu, Pb, benzene, and bacterial toxins), or provoked by isoimmune agents (incompatible transfusion), which is not the case in fish.

Note

[1] RBC clearance is a process in which aged erythrocytes are eliminated from the circulation.

4 Hemogram

Part II: White Blood Count (WBC) and Thrombocyte Count (THRC)

The white blood cell count and thrombocyte count involve techniques for the identification, quantification, and morphological evaluation of circulating leukocytes and thrombocytes, respectively. The methods widely used in mammalian clinical hematology are not fully adequate for fish, since the erythrocytes of these animals are nucleated, which makes it impossible to count in the hemocytometer when using Turk's solution as a hemodiluent. As a result, some researchers have adopted the techniques used in bird clinical hematology, adopting the diluents of Natt and Herrick (1952) or Dacie modified by Blaxhall and Daisley (1973) (Hrubec and Smith, 2001). However, fish leukocyte counts performed by these methods are neither consistent nor accurate, and there are studies that confirm these inconsistencies (Tavares-Dias *et al.*, 2002; Ishikawa *et al.*, 2008; Pádua *et al.*, 2009). Therefore, the most suitable protocols for total leukocyte and thrombocyte counts in the blood in fish are conducted by indirect methods using the erythrocyte count along with total leukocyte and thrombocyte counts (Pitombeira and Martins, 1966; Hrubec and Smith, 1998).

Soon after collecting the blood, smears are made on slides (Fig. 4.1). The remaining blood in the needle or first drops in the tip of the syringe can be used, which is free of anticoagulant. The blood smears would be of good quality, and the blood cells are free of changes caused by the storage of blood and by anticoagulant. The last can alter the permeability of the cell membrane, compromising the staining process.

Procedure

1. The slides must be new, clean, and degreased and always handled by the sides. Two smears should be made for each animal. Even new slides, recently purchased, should be cleaned. There are various products for the preparation of slides. The slides are placed in appropriate detergent solutions for at least 24 h. Afterward, the slides are rinsed in running water for complete removal of the cleaning solutions. They are then placed in a container with alcohol-ether (1:1). The slides are then removed with tweezers and dried with lint-free cotton cloth.

2. The first drops of blood from the needle (without anticoagulant) are placed at the end of the slide (for each slide).

3. A slide with the corners rounded (Fig. 4.1) is placed on the sample slide in front of the droplet at an angle of 45°, which can vary with the viscosity of the blood, and it is slowly moved forward so that the blood is spread uniformly. The thickness of the blood film will depend on the angle of the smearing slide.

4. A rapid sliding movement is used so that the blood spreads in a thin uniform film on the slide.

5. A good preparation should show: head, body, tail, and side margins.

6. The blood film should not be too thin (erythrocytes very far apart) or thick (erythrocytes touching or overlapping).

7. After making the smear, forming a monolayer of cells, one should never blow on the slide or warm the slide for faster drying. The correct way to speed up drying is to shake

© Maria José Ranzani-Paiva, Santiago Benites de Pádua and Marcos Tavares-Dias 2026.
Methods for Haematological Analysis in Fish (Maria José Ranzani Paiva *et al.*)
DOI: 10.1079/9781836991762.0004

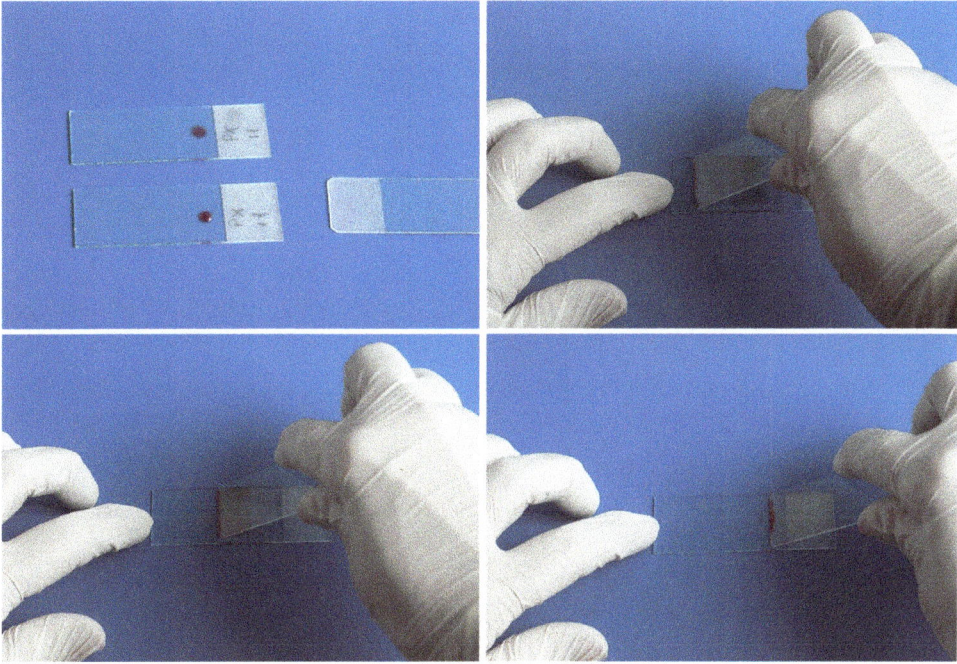

Fig. 4.1. Preparation of blood smears after collecting blood. (Figure author's own.)

the slide in the air. A hairdryer or fan can also be used. Hold the slide by the sides, so as not to warm it with the warmth of the hand.

8. The slide should be labeled with a regular pencil, writing the identification on frosted end of slide or thickest part of the smear or using a sticker. When using stickers, care must be taken at the time of staining so as not to erase the label; if that happens, the slide label must be memorized and replaced. Melted paraffin can be used to impermeabilize the label, before staining.

9. The blood smears should be stained preferably just after preparation or, if not possible, within 30 days with good storage conditions.

Blood Smear Staining

In all stainings, the cell structures with affinity for methylene blue are called basophilic (stained blue); those with affinity for azure are called azurophilic, stained purple (metachromasia); those that have an affinity for the eosin are called acidophilic or eosinophilic (stained orange) and structures which have affinity for the complex mixture are called neutrophilic (stained salmon color).

The stainings used in hematology are panoptic or staining according to Romanowsky. This author devised a method in which a mixture of eosin and methylene blue dyes is prepared. According to the proportion of these salts, these mixtures were named according to their authors: Leishman, Wright, May-Grünwald, and Giemsa, among others. These stains are prepared in methanol, and so the methylene blue is oxidized, resulting in various 'methylene azures.' Thus, this stain is an alcoholic solution of novel compounds called eosin, methylene blue, and azure.

The stains used should be of good quality so as not to compromise cell differentiation.

Staining according to Rosenfeld (1947) is as follows:

Stock stain solution (MMG)
Eosin methylene blue (May-Grünwald) 0.53g
Eosin methylene blue (Giemsa)......... 0.97g

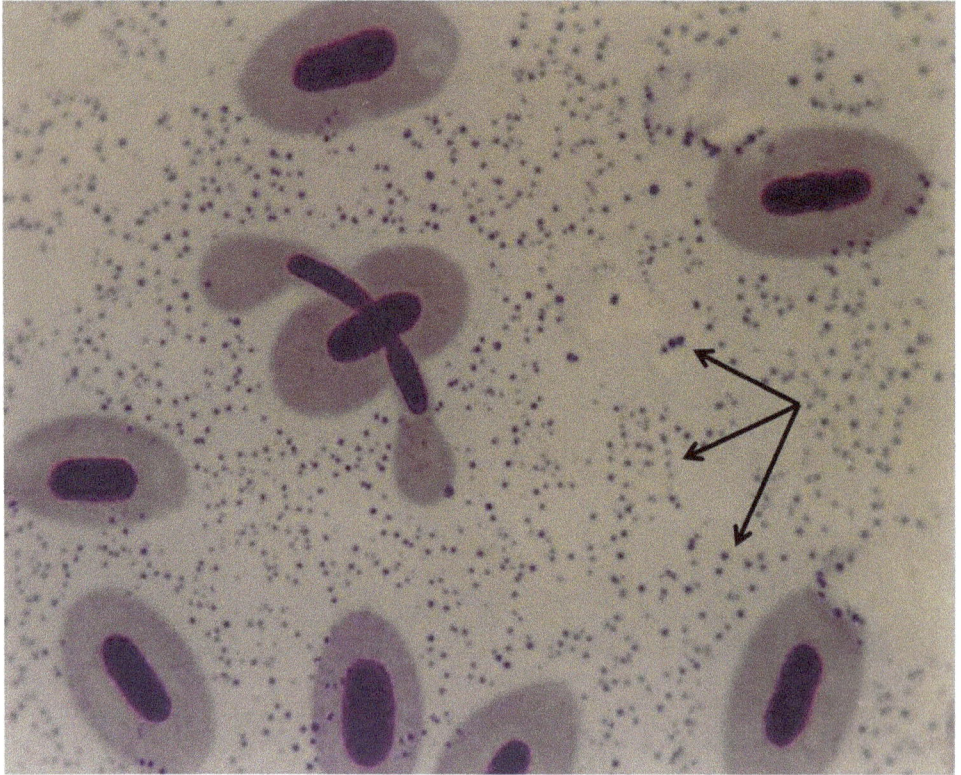

Fig. 4.2. Formation of precipitate of stain (arrows) – small blue points spread throughout the smear. (Figure author's own.)

Methanol ACS .... 1000.0 mL

Observed: Methanol should be of high quality (ACS); otherwise, it can interfere with the quality and effectiveness of the stain. After preparation of the stain, it will be allowed to stand for at least 3 days before use and then always filtered when necessary (formation of precipitate). Care must be taken with the use of methanol, because acute exposure by inhalation causes irritation of the mucous membranes of the respiratory tract, headache, fatigue, insomnia, vertigo, tremors, ringing in the ears, blurred vision, double vision, and blindness. Contact with the skin causes irritation and itchy skin, dermatitis, and eczema. If ingested, it causes serious intoxication manifested by nausea, vomiting, diarrhea, abdominal pain, and neuropsychic and hemodynamic disturbances, which can lead to death.

It is a widely used method for fish, because it is fast, since it uses the two stains, May-Grünwald and Giemsa, in a single solution, saving time in staining.

2. Procedure

1. Cover the smear with ten drops of stain for 3-5 min.
2. Place on the stain the same amount of buffered water (about pH 7.0 and slightly alkaline) or distilled water recently boiled at room temperature, mix with glass or metal rod, and wait for 10 min. It is necessary to test the staining time for the best results. At this point, the salts contained in the alcoholic solution become ionized, and these, once ionized, begin to stain the cellular structures.

Important: Never blow to mix the staining solution/water. The breath contains carbon dioxide that can change the pH of the solution and affect the staining. Care must also be taken when mixing the solution with a rod, not touching the cell layer to avoid damaging the smear.

3. Rinse slide in running water, dry, and examine the slide under a light microscope at 1000×;
4. Avoid staining in a very ventilated environment, which can cause the evaporation of the stain, forming a precipitate on the slides (Fig 4.2.). The formation of precipitate can be avoided by covering the slide with a Petri dish lid. In the case of precipitation of the stain, one option is to immerse the slides quickly (seconds) in methanol and rinse immediately in running water for a few seconds.

This staining is also valid for counting micronuclei in toxicology studies (Kirschbaum *et al.*, 2009; Seriani *et al.*, 2012; Seriani and Ranzani-Paiva, 2012).

Staining using Rosenfeld modified according to Tavares-Dias and Moraes (2003) is as follows:

Stock solution of May-Grünwald-Giemsa (MGG) stain
Eosin methylene blue
(May-Grünwald).........1.0g
Eosin methylene blue (Giemsa)........... 1.0g
Eosin methylene blue (Wright) 0.5g
Methanol ACS. .... 1000.0 mL

Buffer for blood smears (pH 6.8–7.0)
Monobasic potassium phosphate
(KH_2PO_4) 1.63g
Dibasic sodium phosphate (Na_2HPO_4)
.... 3.20g
Distilled water (q.s.p.) .... 1000.0 mL

3. Procedure

1. The smear should be well dry.
2. Cover all the smears with stain for 1-3 min.
3. Dilute with phosphate buffer, pH 6.8-7.0, or distilled water of good quality (add to cover whole slide, without spilling the stain), mix, and let stand for 7-15 min.

4. Next, rinse the slide in running water, and dry and examine the slide under a light microscope at 1000×.
5. If precipitate from the stain forms on the smear, immerse the slides quickly in methanol, so as not to lose all staining, and rinse immediately in running water.

Staining by Giemsa method
Eosin methylene blue
(Giemsa)..................... 8.0g
Glycerol ACS .... 500 mL
Methanol ACS (pH 6.8)
(q.s.p.)...................... 1000 mL

Giemsa is a mixture of azure II and eosin azure. Its use for staining blood smears of fish is indicated for the study of hemoparasites, such as *Trypanosoma*, *Cryptobia*, hemogregarines, and rickettsial agents, which will be discussed at the end of this chapter. In addition, some investigators also use this stain for quantification of micronuclei, where it is not effective in staining granulocytic leukocytes.

4. Procedure

1. Fix the smear with methanol ACS for 3–5 min and air-dry the slide.
2. Dilute the stain with distilled water of good quality, at one to two drops per 1 mL, and mix.
3. Cover the smear with this mixture and let stand for 30–60 min.
4. Next, rinse the smear in running water, dry, and examine the slide under a light microscope at 1000×.
5. If precipitate from the stain forms on the smear, immerse the slides quickly in methanol, so as not to lose all staining, and rinse immediately in running water.
6. In the presence of hemoparasites, it is necessary to make a permanent slide mounted with Canada balsam or similar resin and coverslip and to follow the guidelines for parasitological studies.

Staining according to Leishman
Leishman powder................................ 8.0g
Methanol ACS (pH 6.8)..................1000.00

This stain is a mixture of eosin methylene blue and eosin methylene violet and blue dissolved in methanol. It is one of the most used methods in hematological practices, even in fish because of its technical simplicity and rapidity, in which it stains the different elements in blood. However, for fish, this stain does not always offer good results in differentiating the various types of leukocytes.

5. Procedure

1. Dry the smear.
2. Cover the whole smear with 0.2% Leishman stain in methanol (counting the number of drops) and wait 5 min.
3. Cover the smear with equal number of drops of water and let stand for 10 min.
4. Next, rinse the slide under running water, dry, and examine the slide under a light microscope at 1000×.

Total White Blood Cells

The total leukocyte count can be determined in a direct manner, diluting the blood with the Natt and Herrick solution (1952), used in the hematology of birds, or with that of Dacie modified by Blaxhall and Daisley (1973), where the leukocytes are counted in the outer grids of a Neubauer chamber.

Natt and Herrick diluent (1952) used for counting WBCs is as follows:

NaCl.................................... 3.88g
Na_2SO_4 .... 2.50 g
$Na_2HPO_4.12H_2O$.................. 2.91 g
KH_2PO_4 .... 0.25 g
Formalin (37%).................... 7.50 cc
Methyl violet 2B.................. 0.10 g
Distilled water q.s.p. ..... 1000.00 mL

Using this diluent, the leukocytes are stained purple and are distinguished from the erythrocytes. This method has the disadvantage of staining the thrombocytes and immatures, easily confused with leukocytes.

The indirect method is performed on stained smears by the erythrocytes-leukocytes ratio. In each smear, 2000 cells are counted (including erythrocytes, leukocytes, and thrombocytes), and among them, it is noted how many leukocytes and thrombocytes appear. By the rule of three, considering the total number of cells counted in the Neubauer chamber, the total number of leukocytes and thrombocytes is calculated (Pitombeira and Martins, 1966; Hrubec and Smith, 1998).

Calculation of number of total leukocytes by indirect method

Example: In the Neubauer chamber, 2,500,000 cells μL^{-1} were counted. In smear 2000 cells, 100 leukocytes were counted, so then:

2,000 .... 100 (leukocytes)
2,500,000 x

Absolute number of leukocytes:

$$x = \frac{100 \times 2,500,000}{2000} = 1,25,000 \text{ cells } \mu L^{-1}$$

White Blood Cell Differential or Formula

The differential WBC consists of determining the proportions of different types of leukocytes: neutrophils, eosinophils, basophils, special granulocytic cells (SGCs), lymphocytes, monocytes, and other cells of the leukocyte series.

Peripheral blood cytology is generally studied in blood smears prepared on a

---

Causes of error
- Use of blood with partial clotting.
- Making blood smear with too much blood (thick) or too little blood (thin).
- Poorly made smear, with irregular distribution of cells.
- Slide dirty, greasy, and/or exposed to sun in field collections or exposed to insects (flies and ants).
- Fixation of smear with methanol before staining.
- Blowing on the mixture of stain and water on the smear with pipette.
- Not careful in mixing the stain/water solution with rod, possibly removing the nuclei from the cells.
- Not careful in rinsing the smear with methanol to remove precipitate, possibly destaining the smear completely.

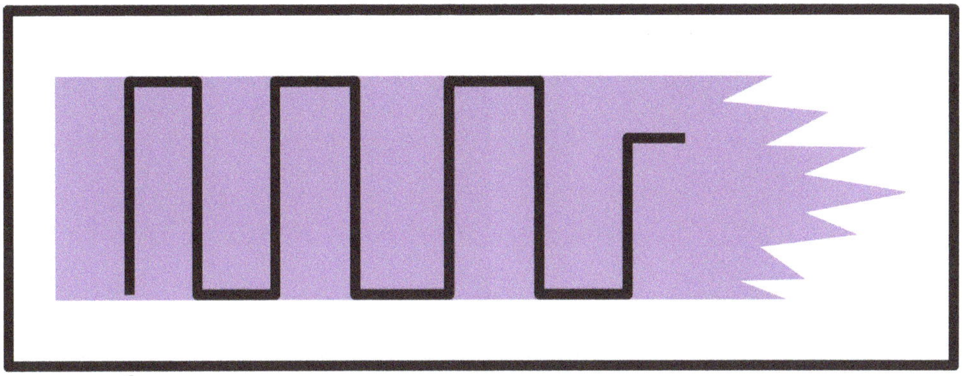

Fig. 4.3. Procedure for total and differential leukocyte counts, total thrombocyte and erythroblast counts, and study of hemoparasites. (Figure author's own.)

good-quality microscope slide. Thus, the cells are so distributed that it facilitates the observation of their structures. Therefore, careful examination of the smear is one of the best ways to study cytomorphological elements and blood parasites as well. In addition, it provides the experienced observer with a good idea of hemoglobin concentration and the number of blood cells.

Technique for differential WBC

1. Prepare two or more blood smears.
2. Stain using the appropriate method.
3. On the microscope, use the oil immersion objective (100×) and classify at least 200 leukocytes. In some studies, when cell differentiation is not very clear, or the smear does not show a very good quality or in leukocytosis (increased number of leukocytes), for example, counting 400 leukocytes is recommended.
4. Counting is done in the body of the smear, moving along the slide in zig-zag manner (Fig. 4.3) because the distribution of the leukocytes on the slide is not uniform. Another way of minimizing errors is to count cells in two smears made from different drops of blood.
5. The number of each element is expressed in percentage, thereby obtaining the relative value. The absolute value is calculated by the rule of three, starting from the total count of leukocytes and the relative value of each element.

6. Examine the morphological features of the leukocytes and note all the degenerative modification that could occur in pathological conditions: alteration of nucleus and alteration of cytoplasm (coloration, vacuolizations, toxic granulations, inclusions, etc.).
7. Be careful with artifacts such as lysed, crenated, crushed and distorted cells, abnormal segmentation of the nucleus due to excess anticoagulant, epithelial cells, 'ghost cells,' and so on.
8. For better conservation of the slides, it is recommended that they be mounted with a coverslip. However, this is not absolutely necessary.

Observed: Smears can be sent to a specialized laboratory to be stained and analyzed. For this, the slides must be identified and wrapped one by one in tissue, so that they do not get scratched, which would make it difficult for analysis and diagnosis. A good way to wrap the slides is to place label against the label because their thickness being sufficient to separate one smear from the other.

Calculation of percentage and total number of leukocytes

The number of leukocytes counted is 200. If, for example, this total included 140 lymphocytes, 30 neutrophils, 20 monocytes, and 10 eosinophils, the percentage of each cell type is listed below:

Lymphocytes = 70%
Neutrophils = 15%
Monocytes = 10%
Eosinophils = 05%

By the preceding calculation, the absolute number obtained is 125,000 leukocytes µL−1. Of these, 70% are lymphocytes, and the calculation is as follows:

125,000 .... 100%

x 70%

Or absolute number of lymphocytes =
$\frac{125,000 \times 70}{100}$ = 87,500 µL−1

The same calculation holds for the other cells. In the end, the sum of the absolute numbers of the different leukocytes should be 125,000.

Interpretation of WBC Count

The leukocytes are often interpreted only by taking into account the differential count in percentage. This is an erroneous practice and can lead to contradictory interpretations. Below is an example of how the same percentage found for leukocytes can mean different absolute numbers.

Example (Jannini and Jannini Filho, 1995):

Two animal problems	(%)	Normal values (%)
Neutrophils	56.0	45.0
Lymphocytes	39.0	50.5
Eosinophils	2.0	1.5
Monocytes	3.0	3.0

Animal 1 – total WBC: 10,000 mL−1
Animal 2 – total WBC: 15,000 mL−1

	Animal 1	Animal 2	Normal
Neutrophils mL−1	5600	8400	2240
Lymphocytes mL−1	3900	5850	6640
Eosinophils mL−1	200	300	250
Monocytes mL−1	300	450	350

Animal 1 – increase in absolute number of neutrophils and decrease in lymphocytes.
Animal 2 – increase in neutrophils, but despite the decrease in percentage of lymphocytes, the absolute number is practically normal.

In addition, some authors refer to the increase (cytosis) or decrease (penia) in numbers of a certain leukocyte, based on the percentage of each cell. This is also wrong, because one cannot speak of lymphocytosis or lymphopenia, for example, without calculating the absolute number of these cells. In Fig. 4.4, we gave two examples of how equal percentage counts can mean different numbers and how different percentage counts can mean equal numbers.

Thrombocytes and Erythroblasts

The calculation done for leukocytes is the same for thrombocytes and erythroblasts.

It is possible, also by this technique, to determine the number of erythroblasts, or immature erythrocytes, which normally appear in the peripheral blood of fish, and which due to some disease can be increased in number. The calculation done for leukocytes is the same for thrombocytes and erythroblasts.

Morpho-Physiological Description of Blood Cells of Fish

The blood cells of fish show wide variation compared with different species, and there can often be variations in the same species, mainly when analyzing the blood cells of sick fish, in which there are pathological changes. The blood cells of fish are the same as those of other vertebrates, with some variations in morphology and perhaps function.

These are the erythrocytes, leukocytes, and thrombocytes. In general, fish have the same types of leukocytes found in other vertebrates, comprising granulocytes, such as neutrophils, heterophils, eosinophils, and basophils, and the agranulocytes, such as monocytes and lymphocytes. However, some species of fish possess some cells that are not found in other vertebrates, such as PAS-positive granular leukocyte (PAS-GL), also known as SGC. In addition, usually in the circulating blood of fish, there are cells in different stages of maturation, which often makes it difficult to determine which type of leukocyte, as a result, they are referred to as immature leukocytes. These cells should be carefully differentiated from erythroblasts, so as not to compromise the leukocyte count.

●	●	●	●	●	50
●	●	●			30
●	●				20
		10			10

Total cells counted 10

●	●	●	●	●	●	●	●	●	●	50
●	●	●	●	●						30
●	●	●								20
						20				100

Total cells counted 20

●	●	●	●	●	52
●	●				25
●					13
		8			100

Total cells counted 20

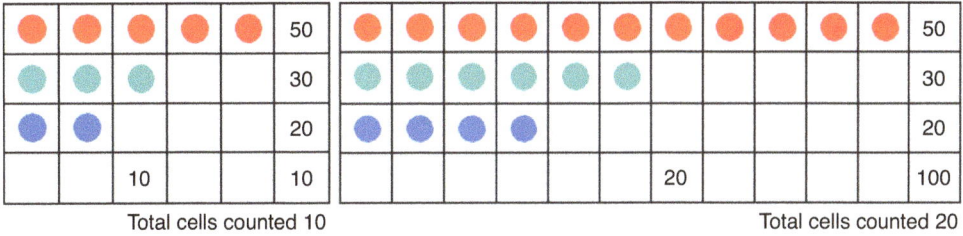

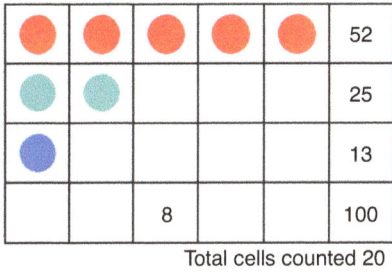

Fig. 4.4. Cytosis or penia? Interpretation of differential leukocyte count is based on percentages. (Figure author's own.)

Erythrocytes

Fish erythrocytes (Fig. 4.5) are true cells, with a nucleus bordered by the nuclear membrane, and their cytoplasm contains several membrane-bounded organelles, which are active and have specific functions. All these materials are enveloped by the semipermeable lipoprotein cytoplasmic membrane. The erythrocytes of fish, amphibians, reptiles, and birds differ from those of mammals, which are anucleated, contain few organelles and have a short lifespan. The function of these cells is the transport of respiratory gases through binding to hemoglobin. Generally, there is a small portion of immature erythrocytes for circulating blood, since in fish, the maturation of these cells can occur in the bloodstream (Satake et al., 2009); in addition, this occurrence can be attributed to the breakdown of homeostasis or to adaptations of biotic and abiotic variables. These cells are very susceptible to oxidative damage because they contain reactive oxygen species, and they are exposed to high oxygen tension, with the consequence of possible alterations in permeability and antigenicity (Wagner et al., 1988; Tavares-Dias and Moraes, 2004). In the different species of fish, one can note morphological variations in these cells, which are generally elliptical with a central nucleus, exhibiting compact chromatin in the mature cells (Fig. 4.5a-f) or loose chromatin in the erythroblasts (Fig. 4.5g-i). Triploid fish (Fig. 4.5e) has larger erythrocytes, and larger nucleus as well, compared with diploid fish (Fig. 4.5f) (Ranzani-Paiva et al., 1998). Blood cells are larger in elasmobranch fish (Fig. 4.5d, i) than in teleost fish (Fig. 4.5a, b, e, h).

Monocytes

Monocytes (Fig. 4.6) are the largest leukocytes in the blood circulation of fish. They have a circular nucleus when young, sometimes with different levels of indentation depending on their maturity (Ranzani-Paiva and Godinho, 1983), where it can show segmentation (Fig. 4.6a), or C shape (Fig. 4.6b) and reniform appearance (Fig. 4.6c) (Silva-Souza et al., 2002). The chromatin is generally purple in color, loose in immature monocytes, and more compact in mature cells. The cytoplasm has a sky-blue color and is free of granulation, but some cytoplasmic vacuoles of different sizes can be observed (Fig. 4.6a, b, d, e, g, h), being generally large and numerous in activated cells (Fig. 4.6i). These leukocytes are the major phagocytes of fish (Ranzani-Paiva, 1995a, b; Silva-Souza et al., 2002; Tavares-Dias and Moraes, 2004; Ranzani-Paiva

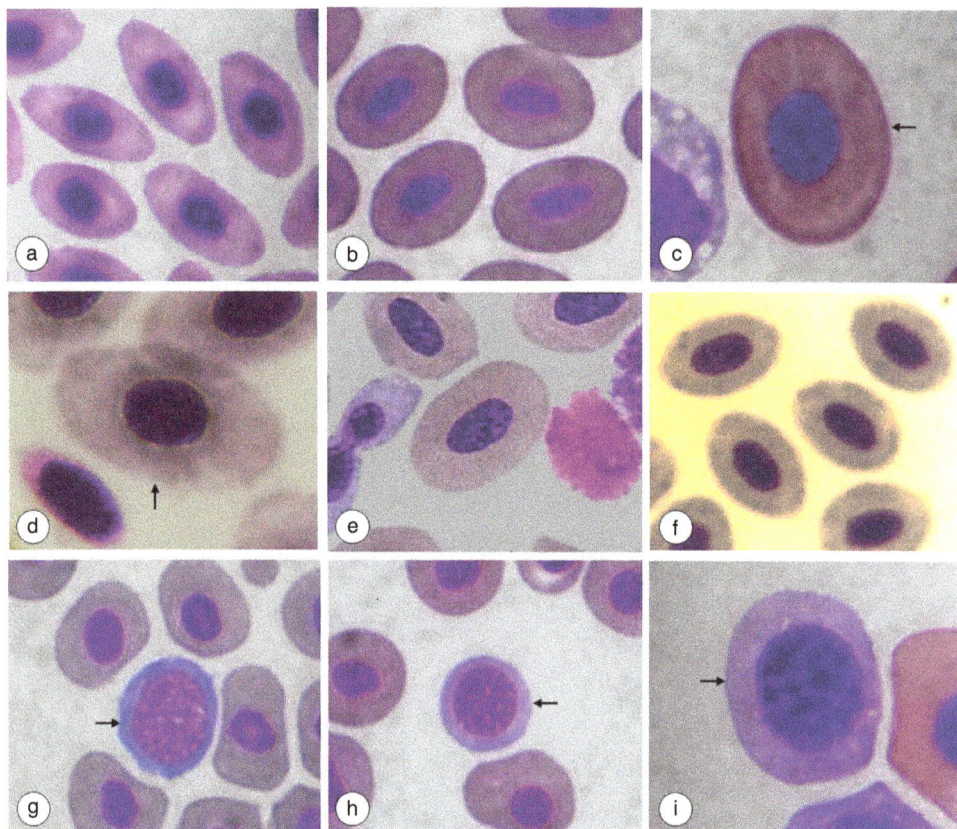

Fig. 4.5. Mature erythrocytes observed in blood smears of tucunaré, *Cichla temensis* (a – Tavares-Dias *et al.*, 2011); pacu, *Piaractus mesopotamicus* (b); Ocellate River stingray, *Potamotrygon motoro* (c – Pádua *et al.*, 2010); nurse shark, *Ginglymostoma cirratum* (d – Napoleão, 2007); rainbow trout, *Oncorhynchus mykiss* triploid (e); and diploid (f). Erythroblasts observed in blood of channel catfish, *Ictalurus punctatus* (g); tuvira, *Gymnotus* aff. *inaequilabiatus* (h); and Ocellate River stingray (i). 1000 × magnification.

et al., 2004) and have the ability to migrate from blood vessels through the mechanism, called diapedesis, to the inflammatory focus by means of chemotaxis during infectious or artificially induced processes (Petric, 2000; Belo *et al.*, 2005; Martins *et al.*, 2009; Santos *et al.*, 2009), thereby becoming macrophages.

Lymphocytes

Lymphocytes are the smallest leukocytes found in circulating fish blood and most abundant in most species. They are characterized by a high nucleus-cytoplasm ratio, with basophilic cytoplasm, free from granulation (Fig. 4.7a-i) (Tavares-Dias *et al.*, 1999). They may be circular or irregular in shape, with numerous cytoplasmic projections (Fig. 4.7c, d, f, g-i). In some species, large, medium, and small lymphocytes can be observed (Ranzani-Paiva, 1996; Veiga *et al.*, 2002). This size variation is possibly related to the maturation stage of the leukocyte, since in the larger cells, chromatin stains light purple and is looser compared with the small lymphocytes. Moreover, these differences may also be related to different populations of lymphocytes, since these are responsible for humoral as well as cellular immunity of the animal, showing different sub-populations (Pádua *et al.*, 2009). Lymphocytes

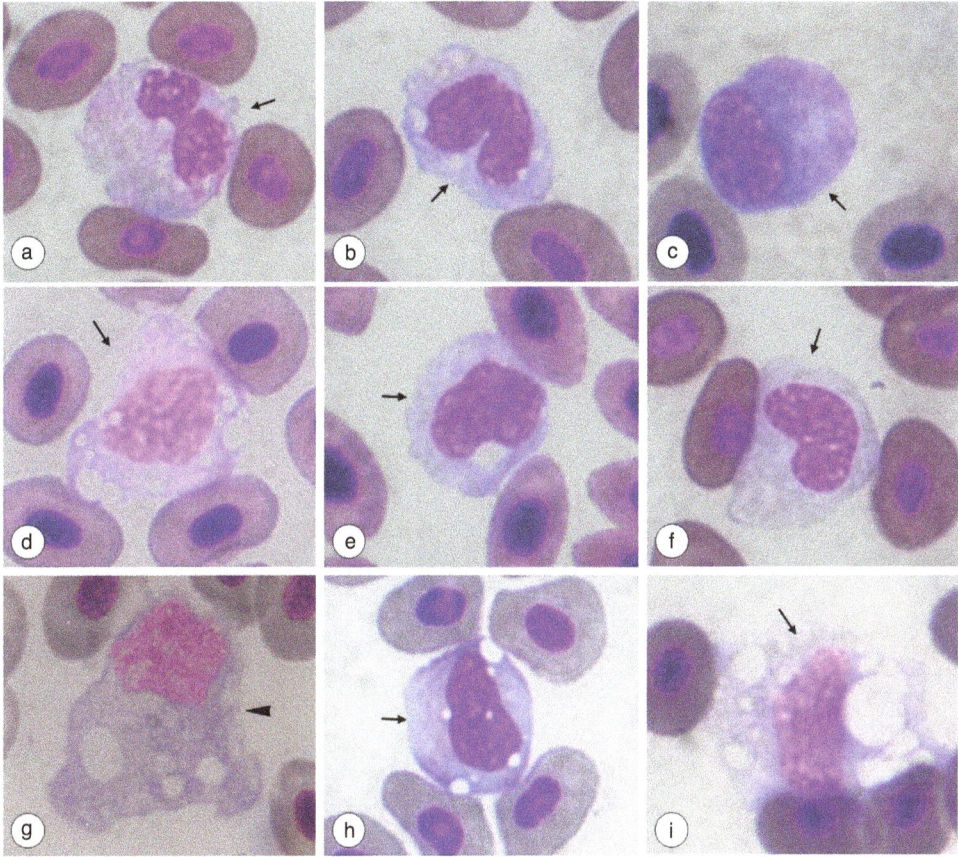

Fig. 4.6. Monocytes observed in blood smears of duckbill catfish, *Sorubim lima* (a); pacu, *Piaractus mesopotamicus* (b); tambaqui, *Colossoma macropomum* (c); pacu-manteiga, *Mylossoma duriventre* (d); tucunaré, *Cichla temensis* (e – Tavares-Dias *et al.*, 2011); piranha, *Serrasalmus* sp. (f), curimbatá, *Prochilodus lineatus* (g – Jensch Jr, 2002); channel catfish, *Ictalurus punctatus* (h); and tilapia, *Oreochromis niloticus* (i). Staining with MGGW (a-f, h, i) and Rosenfeld (g). 1000 × magnification.

are responsible for the recognition of antigens and the mounting of immune response, being produced in lymphoid organs such as the thymus and spleen (Ranzani-Paiva, 2007).

PAS-Positive Granular Leukocyte or Special Granulocytic Cell

The PAS-positive granular leukocyte is a blood cell whose function, to date, has not been elucidated, where it has been called SGC by Ribeiro (1978). However, Barber and Westterman (1975) described the cytochemical peculiarity of this cell in relation to its Periodic acid-Schiff

(PAS) staining, called as PAS-positive granular leukocyte (Fig. 4.8). This characteristic was later observed in cytochemical studies of blood cells of Brazilian fish, which will be discussed in Chapter V. These cells have the ability to migrate to the inflammatory focus in experimentally induced processes, but its participation in these reactions is not known (Martins *et al.*, 2009).

In studies with the barred sorubim, *Pseudoplatystoma reticulatum*, naturally infested by the ciliated protozoan *Ichthyophthirius multifiliis*, great migration of these leukocytes to the inflammatory focus was observed, where the cells were covered by the protozoa stained with PAS. They are large granulocytes

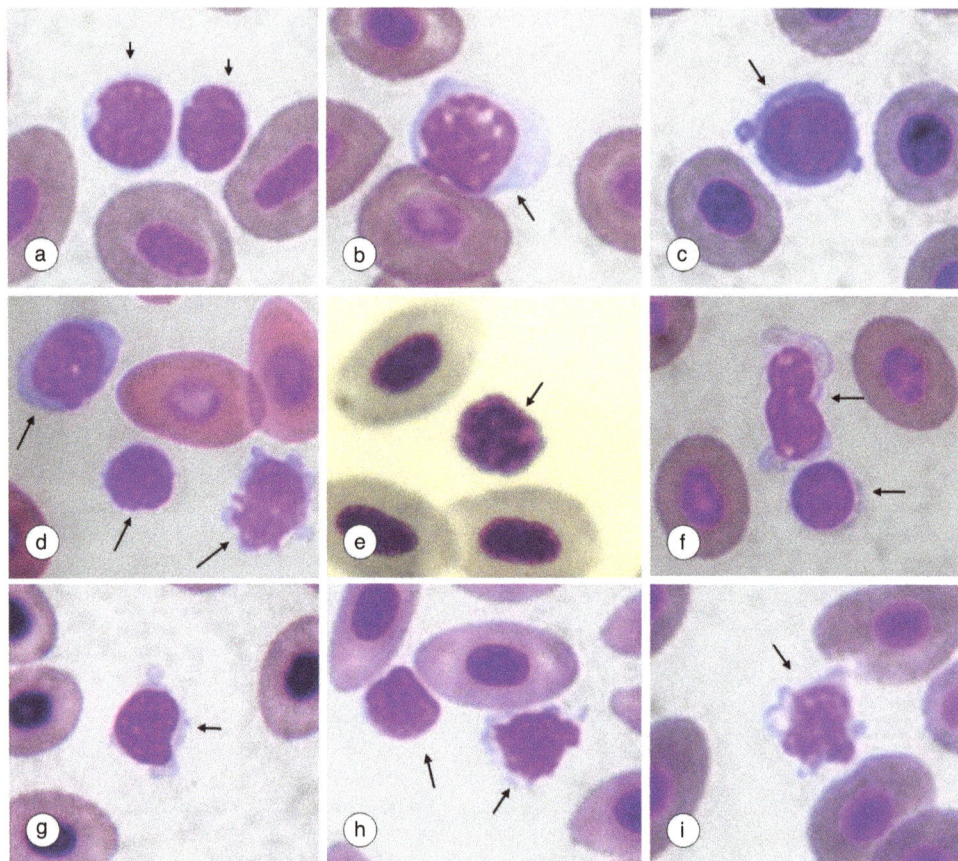

Fig. 4.7. Lymphocytes observed in blood smears of pacu, *Piaractus mesopotamicus* (a); piranha, *Serrasalmus* sp. (b); channel catfish, *Ictalurus punctatus* (c); pirarara, *Phractocephalus hemioliopterus* (d); rainbow trout, *Oncorhynchus mykiss* (e); duckbill catfish, *Sorubim lima* (f); hybrid surubim, *Pseudoplatystoma reticulatum × P. corruscans* (g); tucunaré, *Cichla temensis* (h – Tavares-Dias *et al.*, 2011); and tilapia, *Oreochromis niloticus* (i). Staining with MGGW (a-d, f-h) and Rosenfeld (e, i). 1000× magnification.

with a generally eccentric nucleus located at the periphery of the cell, often with compact chromatin (Fig. 4.8a-i); however, cells with loose chromatin can also be seen in circulating blood (Fig. 4.8d). Its cytoplasm is filled with neutral round granulation, which is not colored by acid or basic stains. Therefore, the cytoplasm is generally white in color and may be slightly basophilic in immature cells (Fig. 4.8d). Since its granulation is extensive, it sometimes seems that the cell is filled with vacuolization (Fig. 4.8c, h); therefore, when analyzing morphological alterations in blood cells, this physiological characteristic should be considered.

Neutrophils

Neutrophils are the main cells responsible for defending the body against bacterial infections, where they phagocytose bacteria. They usually have a round shape (Fig. 4.9a), occasionally having cytoplasmic projections (Fig. 4.9g) or even irregular shapes (Fig. 4.9b, h). The nucleus stains purple colour and has a round shape in immature cells (Pádua *et al.*, 2009) (Fig. 4.9a). It can be oval (Fig. 4.9b), irregular (Fig. 4.9c), reniform (Fig. 4.9d), C-shaped (Fig. 4.9f), and occasionally segmented (Fig. 4.9h, i), depending on cell maturation stage. The cytoplasm has fine neutrophilic

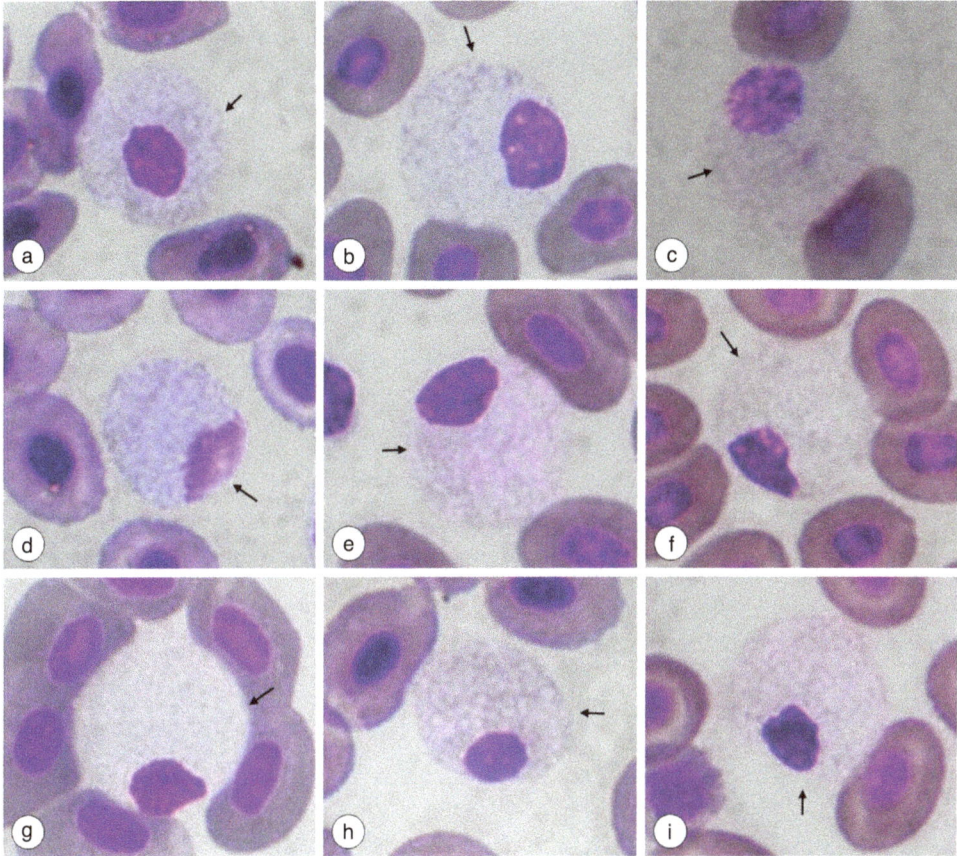

Fig. 4.8. PAS-positive granular leukocyte (PAS-GL), also known as special granulocytic cell (SGC), observed in blood smears of jaraqui, *Semaprochilodus insignis* (a); channel catfish, *Ictalurus punctatus* (b); hybrid surubim, *Pseudoplatystoma reticulatum × P. corruscans* (c); cuiú-cuiú, *Oxydoras niger* (d); pacu, *Piaractus mesopotamicus* (e); duckbill catfish, *Sorubim lima* (f); tambaqui, *Colossoma macropomum* (g); pacu-manteiga, *Mylossoma duriventri* (d); and piranha, *Serrasalmus* sp. (i). Staining with MGGW. 1000× magnification. (Figure author's own.)

granulation (Ranzani-Paiva and Godinho, 1983) and may be salmon colored in some fish (Veiga *et al.*, 2002) (Fig. 4.9d); occasionally, the presence of small cytoplasmic vacuoles can be observed in mature cells (Fig. 4.9f, h). Some neutrophil populations exhibit prominent eosinophilic granules and resemble avian and reptile heterophils as well as 'fine eosinophilic granulocytes' of cartilaginous fish (Clauss *et al.*, 2008).

Heterophils

Heterophils are cells with the same function as neutrophils but constitute different leukocyte varieties (Claver and Quaglia, 2009). These cells are found only in some species of teleost fish, such as those belonging to the genera *Brycon* (Tavares-Dias *et al.*, 2008), *Salminus* (Pádua *et al.*, 2009), *Hoplosternum* (Tavares-Dias and Barcellos, 2005), and in the elasmobranchs (Napoleão, 2007; Pádua *et al.*, 2010). Some fish can simultaneously have neutrophils and heterophils in circulating blood. These cells have oval nuclei, which can be central or eccentric, with compact chromatin. Its cytoplasm may show fine neutrophilic granulation with some very basophilic granules (Fig. 4.10a) or robust acidophilic granulation, as seen with the staining of eosinophil granules (Fig. 4.10b, c). Since they

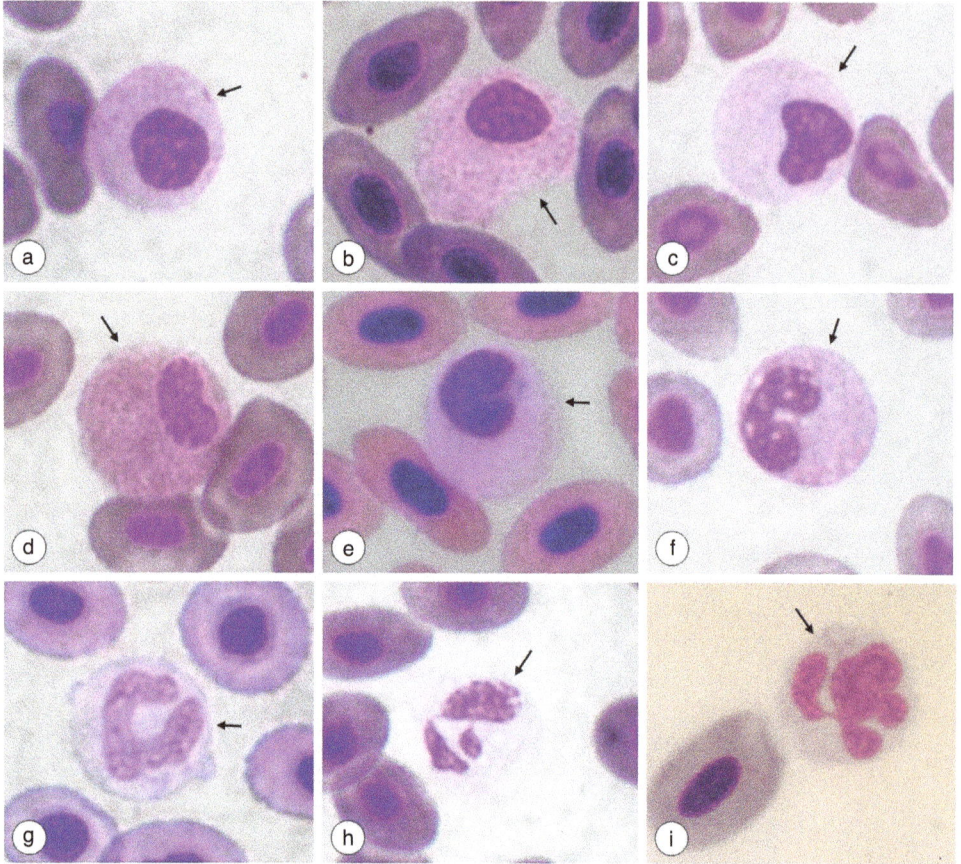

Fig. 4.9. Neutrophils observed blood smears of tuvira, *Gymnotus* aff. *inaequilabiatus* (a); tucunaré, *Cichlas temensis* (b); jurupensém, *Surubim lima* (c); pacu, *Piaractus mesopotamicus* (d); dourado, *Salminus brasiliensis* (e); hybrid surubim, *Pseudoplatystoma reticulatum* × *P. corruscans* (f); cuiú-cuiú, *Oxydoras niger* (g); tilapia, *Oreochromis niloticus* (h); and rainbow trout, *Oncorhynchus mykiss* (i). Staining with MGGW (a-g) and Rosenfeld (h, i). 1000 × magnification. (Figure author's own.)

are phagocytes, the presence of small vacuoles in their cytoplasm is common (Fig. 4.10b, c).

Eosinophils

Eosinophils exhibit wide variation in shape, granules, and size as well. They may be large leukocytes (Fig. 4.11a-e), but generally small eosinophils (Fig. 4.11d-i) are predominant in different fish species. The nucleus has purple-stained chromatin, is round or oval, and may occasionally show segmentation (Fig. 4.11a). The cytoplasm is hyaline or slightly basophilic and contains a varied amount of eosinophilic staining. The granules may be in the shape of crystalloid or rounded rods, similar to those seen in human eosinophils (Claver and Quaglia, 2009). Mature cells (Fig. 4.11a, d, f, h) have granulation-filled cytoplasm, whereas young eosinophils have few cytoplasmic granules (Fig. 4.11i). Round fish (pacu, tambaqui, pirapitinga, and their interspecific hybrids) generally exhibit young eosinophils with small, rod-shaped cytoplasmic granulation (Fig. 4.11i), whereas mature cells have round granules (Fig. 4.11b). The function of eosinophils in fish is still uncertain, although there is evidence of their participation in defense processes against

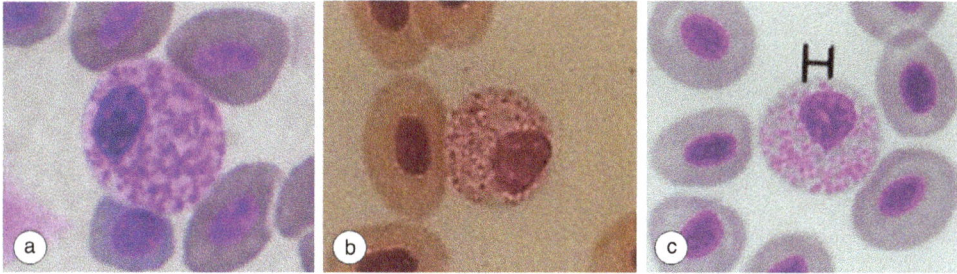

Fig. 4.10. Heterophils observed in blood smears of dourado, *Salminus brasiliensis* (a); curimbatá, *Prochilodus lineatus* (b); and matrinxã, *Brycon amazonicus* (c) (Affonso *et al.*, 2007), exhibiting acidophilic (neutrophilic) and basophilic granulation. Staining with MGGW (a, c) and MMG (b). 1000 × magnification.

parasites (Martins *et al.*, 2004) as observed in other vertebrates. However, there is not always an increase in the number of eosinophils in parasitized fish. Eosinophils circulate for a certain time and migrate to tissues under stimulation of infection/infestation (Ranzani-Paiva, 2007) as demonstrated by Menezes *et al.* (2011), who found severe inflammatory eosinophilic reaction in the stomach of pirarucu infected by *Goezia spinulosa*.

Basophils

Basophils are rare leukocytes in the circulating blood of most fish species (Clauss *et al.*, 2008) but are common in some fish such as catfish belonging to the genus *Pseudoplatystoma*. They may be irregular cells (Fig. 4.12a, e, f) or rounded (Fig. 4.12b, c) and medium-sized (Fig. 4.12b, c) to small (Fig. 4.12h, i). The nucleus stains purple and can be elongated (Fig. 4.12a), circular (Fig. 4.12f), with a chamfer (Fig. 4.12h) or oval (Fig. 4.12i). Chromatin is loose in immature cells (Fig. 4.12g) and compact with maturation (Fig. 4.12h). The cytoplasm has a varied amount of basophilic granulation, which in some cases may hamper the examination of the nucleus (Fig. 4.12d). As with eosinophils, the number of granules in basophils is related to the degree of cell maturation. In addition, in 'surubins,' immature basophils may also show rod-shaped cytoplasmic granulation (Fig. 4.12g). The role of this leukocyte is not yet elucidated in fish, although there is evidence of its involvement in the process of phagocytosis, especially in

the removal of cell debris (Satake *et al.*, 2009); perhaps for this reason, one can find basophils exhibiting cytoplasmic vacuolization in some fish (Fig. 4.12d).

Immature Leukocytes

Immature leukocytes (Fig. 4.13a-e) are commonly found in the circulation of healthy fish, and the final maturation of these cells can occur in the bloodstream. This physiological capacity for differentiation does not occur in mammals. For this reason, when immature leukocytes are present in fish blood, a false leukemic state is produced (Ranzani-Paiva, 1995a).

Identification of these cells can be hampered by the presence of basophilic erythroblasts (Fig. 4.13d-f), as they are very similar. Satake *et al.* (2009) cite the following criteria that aid in the differentiation of these cells:

1. Appearance of chromatin: basophilic in erythroblasts, generally rough compared with immature leukocytes.
2. Location of nucleus: in basophilic erythroblasts, generally in the center of the cell, while in immature leukocytes, it is located preferentially on cell periphery, with opposite displacement of the cytoplasm.
3. Cell shape: basophilic erythroblasts generally have regular elliptical shape along with the nucleus; in immature leukocytes, the shape of the nucleus may be irregular, round, or reniform.

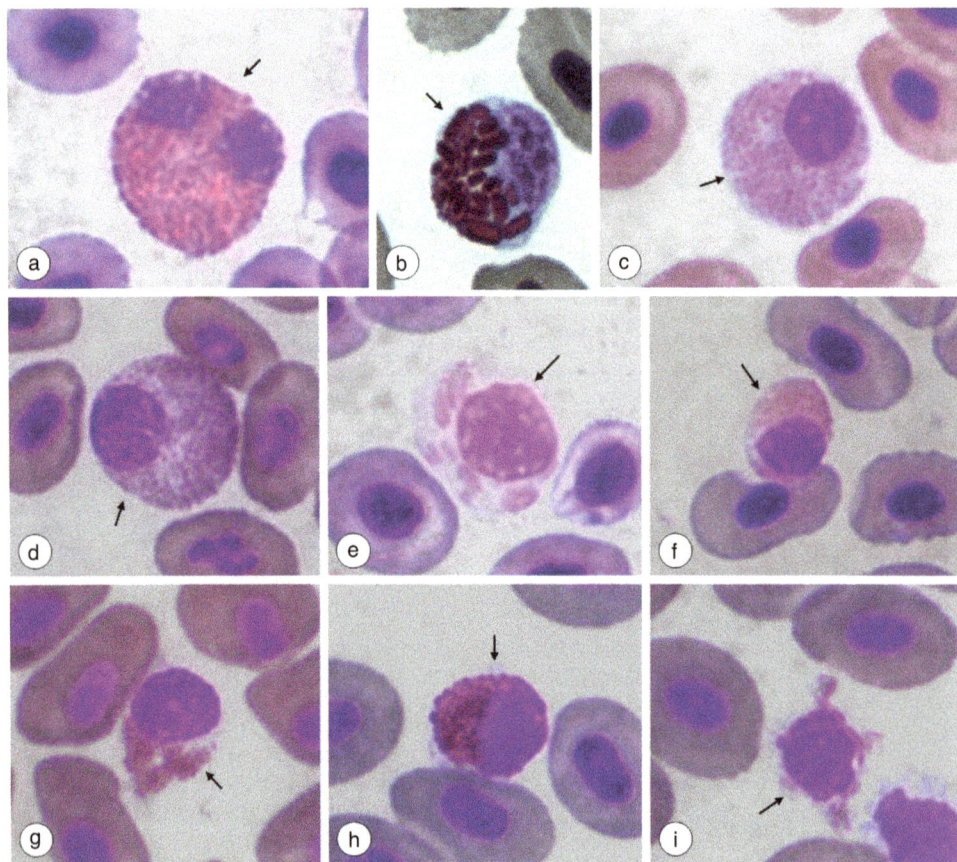

Fig. 4.11. Eosinophils observed in blood smears of 'cuiú-cuiú' *Oxydoras niger* (a); dourado, *Salminus brasiliensis* (b); surubim hybrid, *Pseudoplatystoma reticulatum × P. corruscans* (c); jurupensém, *Surubim lima* (d); jaraqui, *Semaprochilodus insignis* (e); pacu-manteiga, *Mylossoma duriventri* (f); piranha, *Serrasalmus* sp. (g); and pacu, *Piaractus mesopotamicus* (h, i). Staining with MGGW (a, c-i) and Rosenfeld (b) 1000 × magnification. (Figure author's own.)

Thrombocytes

Thrombocytes are not only body defense cells, mainly involving blood coagulation, but also phagocytosis, especially in the removal of cellular debris (Matushima and Mariano, 1996; Tavares-Dias *et al.*, 2007b). In addition, they have the ability to migrate to an inflammatory focus in experimentally induced processes. In most species, they have an elliptical shape, high nucleus-cytoplasm ratio, and hyaline cytoplasm (Fig. 4.14b, d, e, g-i) or exhibit fine acidophilic granulation (Fig. 4.14c, f). The purple-colored nucleus has the same shape as the cell. It shows loose chromatin in immature cells (Fig. 4.14a – dashed arrow) and compacts at maturation. Occasionally, cytoplasmic vacuolation can be observed in these cells, possibly related to phagocytic activity.

Study of Blood Parasites

The parasites mostly found in fish blood are protozoan trypanosomes (Fig. 4.15a-c) and hemogregarines (Fig. 4.15d, e), and Rickettsiae (Fig. 4.15f), along with a variety of viral inclusions and unknown bodies. The investigation

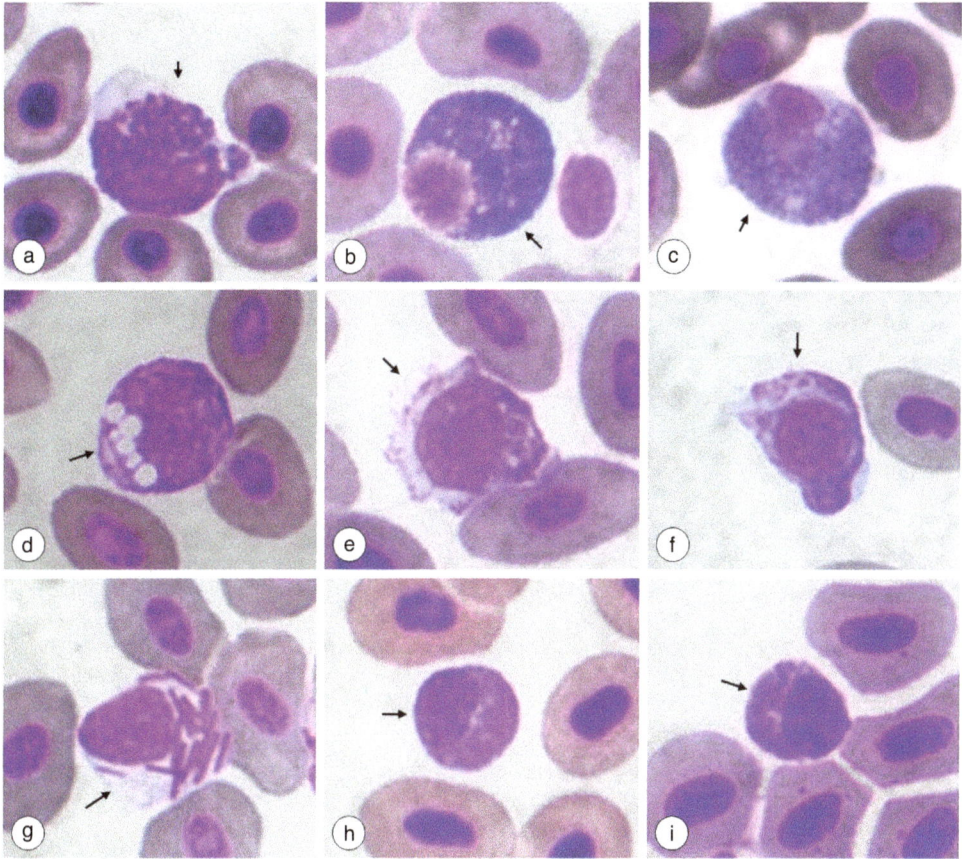

Fig. 4.12. Basophils observed in blood smears of tuvira, *Gymnotus* aff. *inaequilabiatus* (a); pirarara, *Phractocephalus hemioliopterus* (b); tilapia, *Oreochromis niloticus* (c); jurupensém, *Surubim lima* (d); tambacu, *Colossoma macropomum* × *Piaractus mesopotamicus* (e); channel catfish, *Ictalurus punctatus* (f); hybrid surubim, *Pseudoplatystoma reticulatum* × *P. corruscans* (g, h); and dourado, *Salminus brasiliensis* (i). Staining with MGGW. 1000 × magnification. (Figure author's own.)

of these hemoparasites can be performed in the same procedure as differential counting of leukocytes, but for a more accurate investigation, one must look along the edges and tail of the smear, where the parasitized cells and the hemoparasites themselves are concentrated. However, sometimes blood can be contaminated with some parasites that are not necessarily hemoparasites. Among these, it may be common to observe spores of Myxosporidia (Fig. 4.16a–d), which in turn is not the infecting stage for the fish. The observation of these myxosporids in the blood can be attributed to the contamination of the needle at the time of collection of the blood,

as it can break up plasmodia present in the skin and/or musculature. Also, the slide can be contaminated by algae, when the water on the own fish falls carelessly on the slide.

In non-stained blood smears, it is possible, for a while, to visualize the extracellular flagellate protozoa by their active movement. The most appropriate form for fresh parasitological examinations is the examination of a drop of blood between a slide and coverslip (Fig. 4.17). Intracellular parasites are only visible after staining of the cells by routine hematological techniques (Ranzani-Paiva *et al.*, 1997).

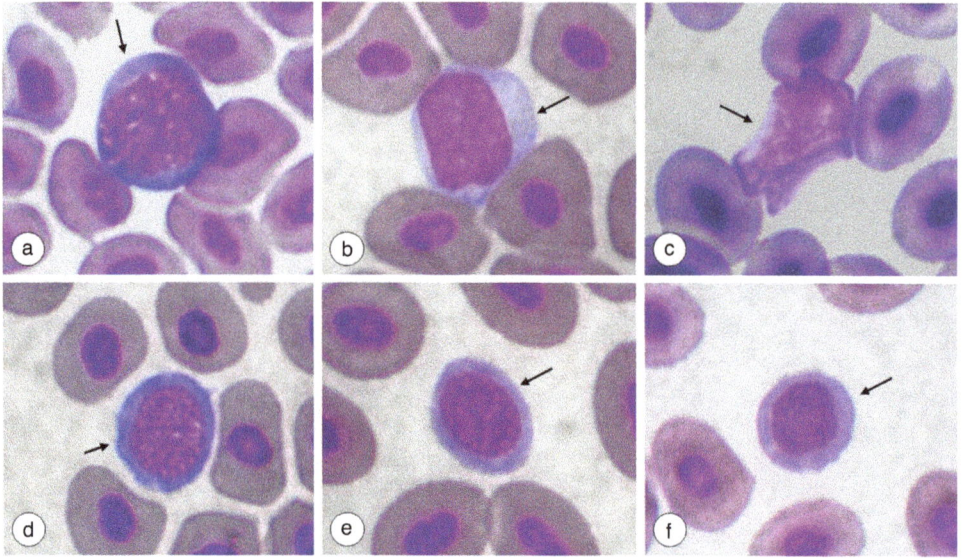

Fig. 4.13. Immature leukocytes observed in blood smears of dourado, *Salminus brasiliensis* (a); hybrid surubim, *Pseudoplatystoma reticulatum* × *P. corruscans* (b); and pacu-manteiga, *Mylossoma duriventri* (c). Basophilic erythroblasts observed in blood smears of channel catfish, *Ictalurus punctatus* (d); pacu, *Piaractus mesopotamicus* (e); and hybrid surubim, *Pseudoplatystoma reticulatum* × *P. corruscans* (f). Staining with com MGGW. 1000 × magnification. (Figure author's own.)

In addition to hemoparasites and other types of parasites that may eventually be found in blood smears, one may see various cytoplasmic inclusions and cells at different stages of degeneration, due to various pathologies, especially those caused by viruses and toxicological agents (Table 4.1). Fig. 4.18 shows some of these inclusions found in Brazilian fish species. Although there is evidence that it is a viral disease, there is no confirmation of the diagnosis so far. Studies of this nature should be increased to understand these anomalies.

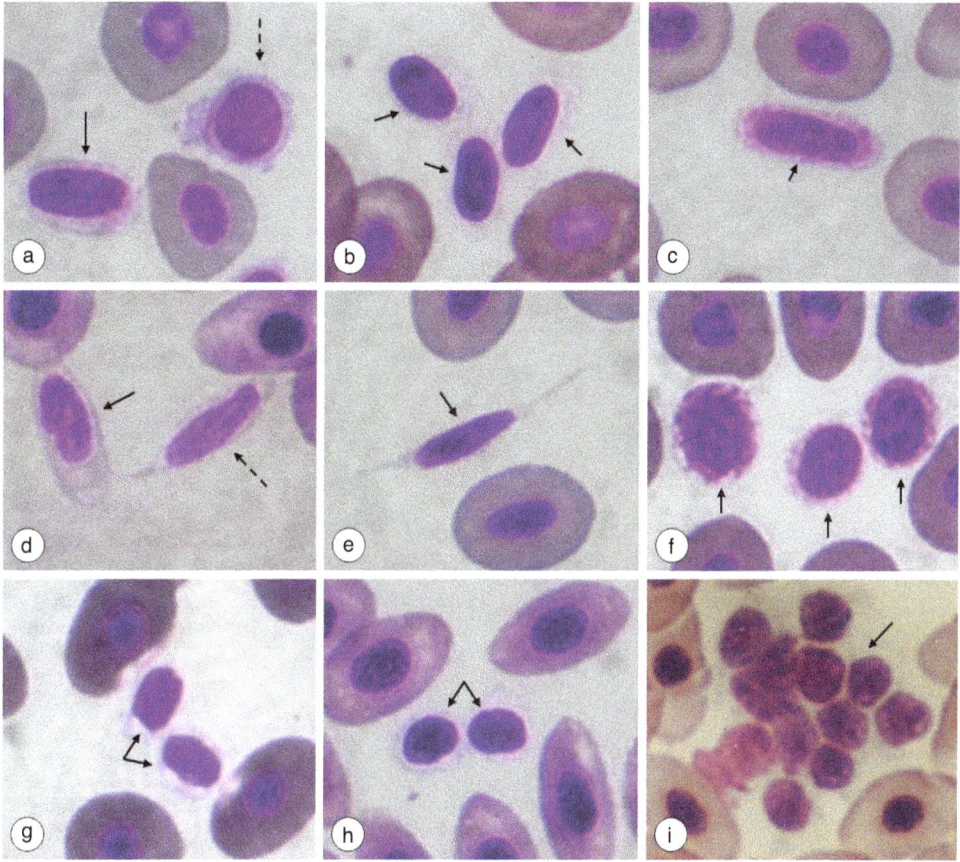

Fig. 4.14. Thrombocytes elliptical (solid arrow) and rounded (dashed arrow) in channel catfish, *Ictalurus punctatus* (a); piranha, *Serrasalmus* sp. (b); thrombocytes exhibiting fine acidophilic granulation in hybrid surubim, *Pseudoplatystoma reticulatum × P. corruscans* (c); thrombocytes elliptical (solid arrow) and fusiform (dashed arrow) in jaraqui, *Semaprochilodus insignis* (d); thrombocytes fusiform in pacu-manteiga, *Mylossoma duriventri* (e); thrombocytes oval exhibiting fine acidophilic granulation in tuvira, *Gymnotus* aff. *inaequilabiatus* (f); thrombocytes with hyaline cytoplasm in tilapia, *Oreochromis niloticus* (g); tucunaré, *Cichlas temensis* (h); and thrombocyte aggregation in tainha, *Mugil platanus* (i – Ranzani-Paiva, 1995a). Staining with MGGW (a-h) and Leishman (i). 1000 × magnification.

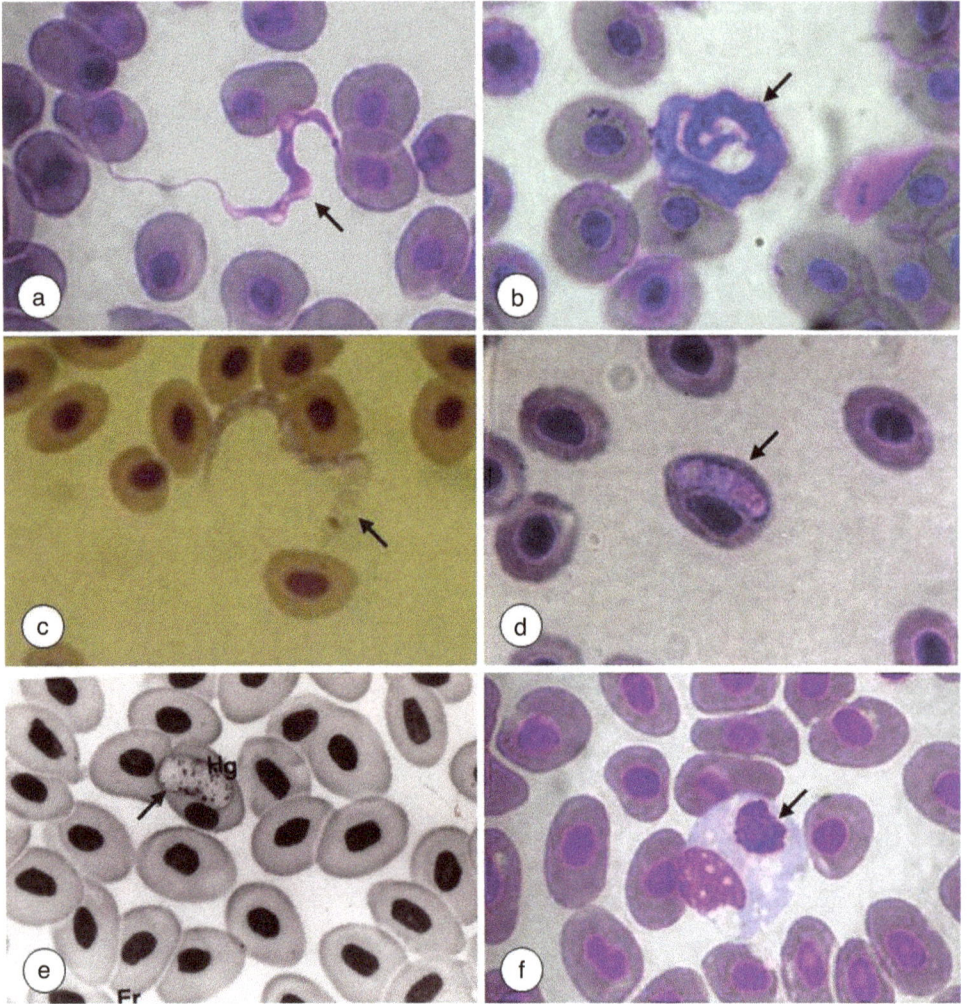

Fig. 4.15. *Trypanosoma* sp. in tuvira, *Gymnotus* aff. *inaequilabiatus* (a); cascudo, *Liposarcus anisitsi* (b); *Trypanosoma platanusi* (c); *Desseria* sp. in tainha, *Mugil platanus* (d); *Haemogregarina* sp. in mussum, *Synbranchus marmoratus* (e); and Anaplasmataceae-like organisms in surubim hybrid, *Pseudoplatystoma reticulatum* × *P. corruscans* (f). 1000 × magnification. (Figure author's own.)

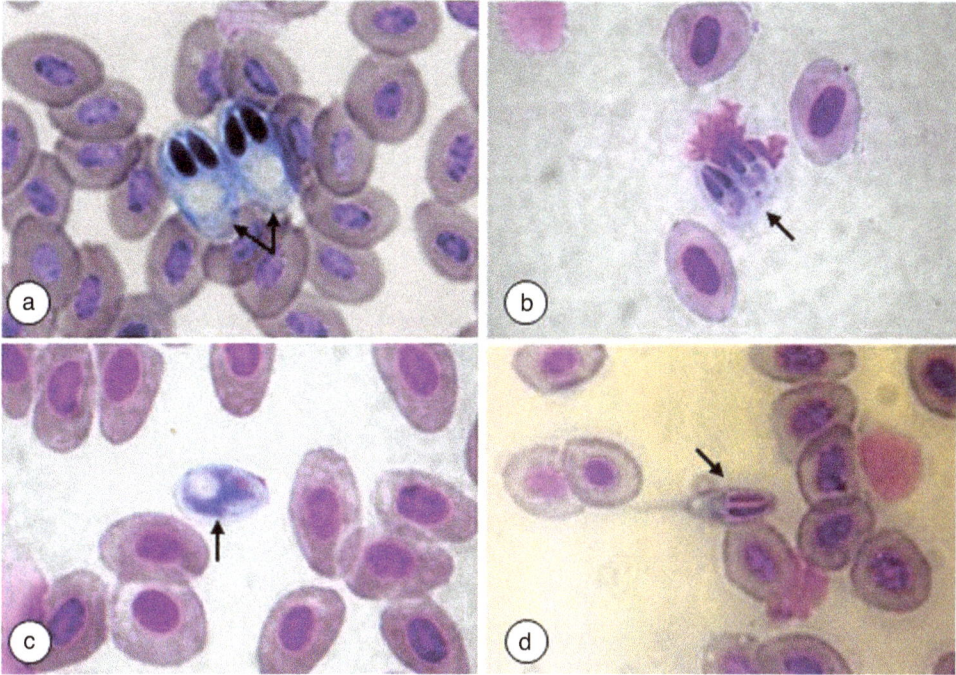

Fig. 4.16. Spores of myxosporids in blood smears of fish. *Myxobolus* sp. (a-c) in blood smear of curimbatá, *Prochilodus lineatus* (a), jaraqui, *Semaprochilodus insignis* (b), and hybrid surubim, *Pseudoplatystoma reticulatum* × *P. corruscans* (c). *Henneguya* sp. in blood smear of curimbatá, *Prochilodus lineatus* (d). 1000 × magnification. (Figure author's own.)

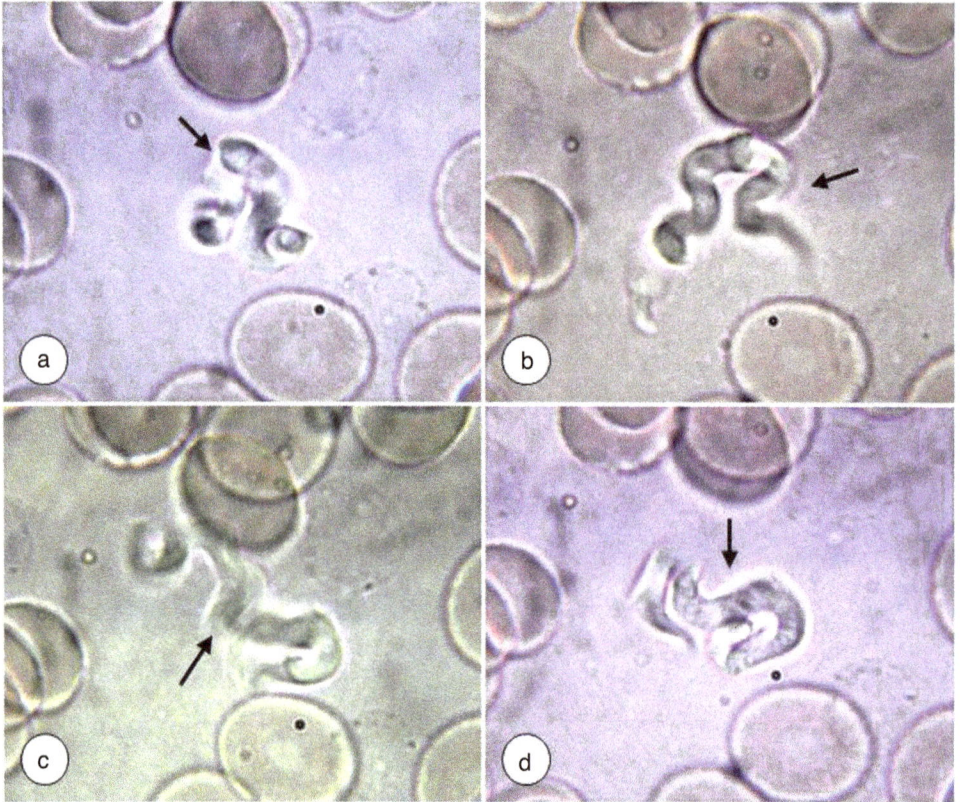

Fig. 4.17. Observation of *Trypanosoma* sp. in direct examination of a drop of blood under a light microscope. 1000 × magnification. (Figure author's own.)

Table 4.1. Lists the main hemoparasites described in the literature on fish. (Table author's own).

Hemoparasites	Taxonomic group	Site of infection	Hosts	References
Anaplasmataceae-like	Rickettsiales	Monocytes	*Pseudoplatysto reticulatus ×P. corruscans*	Ishikawa *et al.* (2011)
Cryptobia acipenseris	Kinetoplastida	Plasma	*Acipenser guldenstadt and A. persicus*	Pazooki and Masoumian (2004)
Cyrilla gomesi	Aipcomplexa	Erythrocytes and plasma	*Synbranchus marmoratus*	Nakamoto *et al.* (1991)
Cyrilla gomesi	Aipcomplexa	Erythrocytes and plasma	*Synbranchus marmoratus*	Diniz *et al.* (2002)
Desseria sp.	Apicomplexa	Erythrocytes and plasma	*Mugil cephalus*	Smit *et al.* (2002)
Haemogregarina acipenser	Apicomplexa	Erythrocytes and plasma	*Acipenser guldenstadt and A. persicus*	Masoumian (2004)

Continued

Table 4.1. Continued

Hemoparasites	Taxonomic group	Site of infection	Hosts	References
Haemogregarina bigemina	Apicomplexa	Erythrocytes and plasma	*Parablennius cornutus*	Davies *et al.* (2003)
Haemogregarina delagei	Apicomplexa	Erythrocytes and plasma	Rajidae	Aragort *et al.* (2005)
Haemogregarina sp.	Apicomplexa	Leukocytes	*Anguilla anguilla*	Orecka-Grabda and Wierzbicka (1998)
Haemogregarina bigemina	Apicomplexa	Erythrocytes	*Lipophrys pholis*	Hayes and Smit (2019)
Haemogregarina daviesensis	Apicomplexa	Erythrocytes	*Lepidosiren paradoxa*	Esteves-Silva *et al.* (2019)
*Myxobolus colossomatis*a	Myxosporea	Plasma	*Colossoma macropomum*	Maciel *et al.* (2011)
Myxobolus sp.a	Myxosporea	Plasma	*Synodontis clarias*	Hassan *et al.* (2007)
Theileria electrophori	Apicomplexa	Erythrocytes, lymphocytes, and plasma	*Electrophorus electricus*	Lainson (2007)
Trypanosoma giganteum	Kinetoplastida	Plasma	Rajidae	Aragort *et al.* (2005)
Trypanosoma platanusi	Kinetoplastida	Plasma	*Mugil platanus*	Ribeiro *et al.* (1996)
Trypanosoma sp.	Kinetoplastida	Plasma	*Clarias gariepus* and *Synodontis clarias*	Hassan *et al.* (2007)
Trypanosoma sp.	Kinetoplastida	Plasma	*Gymnotus* aff. *inaequilabiatus*	Pádua *et al.* (2011)
Trypanosoma sp.	Kinetoplastida	Plasma	*Hypostomus strigaticeps*	Molina *et al.* (2016)
Trypanosoma sp.	Kinetoplastida	Plasma	*Hypostomus* spp.	Molina *et al.* (2016)
Trypanosoma sp.	Kinetoplastida	Plasma	*Gymnotus* aff. *inaequilabiatus* and *Hypostomus albopunctatus*	Molina *et al.* (2016)
Trypanosoma sp.	Kinetoplastida	Plasma	*Carassius auratus*	Corrêa et al. (2016)

aMyxosporeans in blood smears are not enough to consider them as hemoparasites.

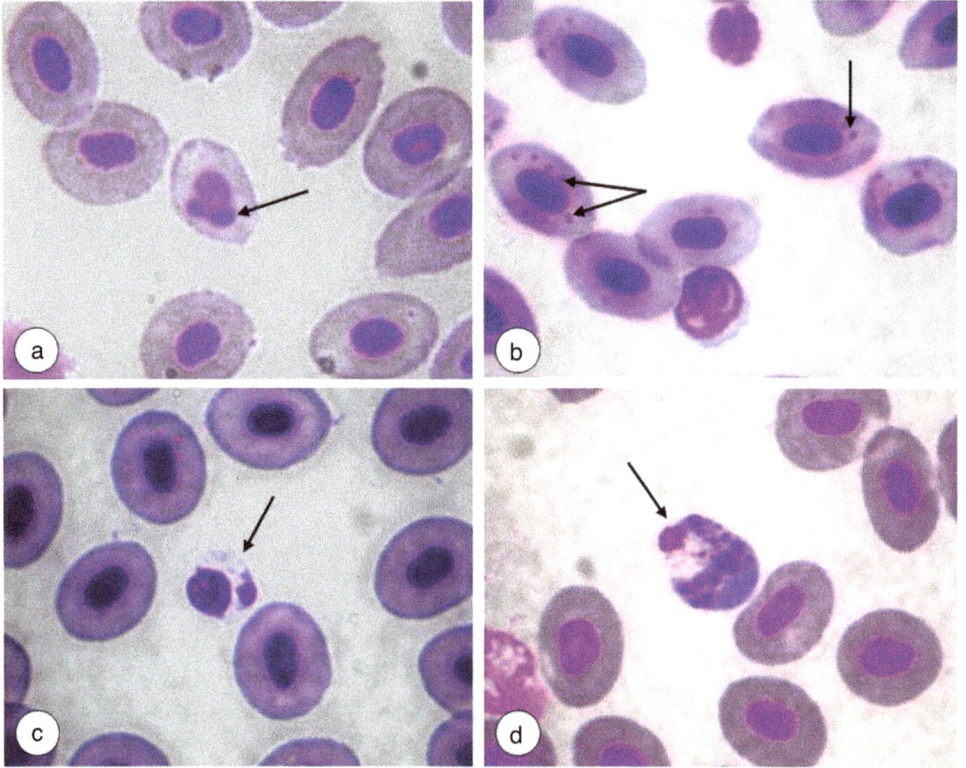

Fig. 4.18. Unidentified inclusions in erythrocytes of curimbatá, *Prochilodus lineatus* (a); tambaqui, *Colossoma macropomum* (b); blood cells in degeneration process (karyorex and vacuolization cytoplasmic) in *Mylossoma duriventri* (c); and hybrid surubim, *Pseudoplatystoma reticulatum* × *P. corruscans* (d). (Figure author's own.)

5 Cytochemical Methods Used for Blood Cells

In general, fish leukocytes show a wide morphological diversity, being made up of different cell types, which display structural heterogeneity often related to the species or the maturation of the cells in the circulatory system. Certain leukocytes are considered to be key mediators in the innate immune response through evolution. These cells confer protection against pathogens by phagocytosis and the action of antibacterial nitrogenous amino acids or enzymes. Most of these products are found in the cytoplasm of leukocytes, being very important in leukocyte physiology and essential for defense. Due to their great importance, their detection by cytochemical methods has developed very much in the studies of fish.

In the case of neutrophilic and eosinophilic granulocytes, enzymes and antibacterial substances are found in specific (secondary) and non-specific (primary or azurophilic) cytoplasmic granules and are involved in the killing of microorganisms after fusion of phagosomes containing foreign material with these granules found in the cytoplasm, forming the phagolysosomes. Enzymes generally have hydrolysis and oxidation functions in granulocytes, but not all can be demonstrated cytochemically. Oxidative enzymes are related to the death of microorganisms by the oxidation and formation of free radicals, and the hydrolytic enzymes, in turn, are important in the digestion of dozens of substances susceptible to their action. In neutrophils and eosinophils, the non-specific granules are abundant in the immature phases, and the specific ones are predominant in the mature phase.

In general, the chemical mechanism of a cytochemical reaction at the tissue or cell level is as follows:

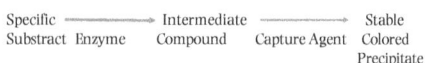

$$\text{Specific Substract} \xrightarrow{\text{Enzyme}} \text{Intermediate Compound} \xrightarrow{\text{Capture Agent}} \text{Stable Colored Precipitate}$$

An incubation medium containing the specific substrate is used, and the appropriate pH and ideal temperature are set for each enzyme, which, in the presence of cofactors or ions and a capture agent, a stable-colored end product is formed. Immediately after the enzymatic action, an intermediate compound is formed which, upon reaction with the capture agent, yields a final colored product, which is essential for light microscope analysis.

In addition to the enzymatic constituents found in the granules of leukocytes, the cytoplasm of these cells contains various chemical substances, such as carbohydrates and lipids (Tavares-Dias, 2006b; Biller and Takahashi, 2018; Cunha *et al.*, 2021). There are cytochemical methods for locating these substances in fish blood cells, which are based on the production of a stained precipitate or the selective dissolution of a dye in lipids. The recognition of cell types, the characterization of the granules present in these cells, the dynamics of their appearance during maturation in the hematopoietic organs, and the role of these leukocyte granules in the various physiological and pathological processes are of great value. This information can be obtained through the application of various classical cytochemical methods, for example, the Periodic acid-Schiff (PAS) reaction for the

Methods for Haematological Analysis in Fish (Maria José Ranzani Paiva *et al.*)
DOI: 10.1079/9781836991762.0005

detection of glycogen and neutral glycoproteins, of Sudan Black B for lipids and membrane lipoproteins and bromophenol blue for proteins in general and for color development with enzymes such as leukocyte peroxidase (myeloperoxidase), esterases, and phosphatases.

The cytochemical methods, in addition to being able to identify the various types of leukocytes, may help to understand the development of these cells and their immunological functions in fish (Ueda et al., 2001; Tripathi et al., 2004; Tavares-Dias, 2006b; Silva et al., 2011; Zhang et al., 2019). In fish, often due to the great morphological variation of leukocytes, the analysis based only on cell morphology after application of the Romanovsky-type mixture may not provide enough information for the identification of these cell populations. This difficulty may render the identification inaccurate, and consequently, the nomenclature adopted for the leukocyte lineages in the numerous known fish species (Tavares-Dias and Moraes, 2004; Pádua and Ishikawa, 2011; Zhang et al., 2019). Thus, the classic hematological stains should also be performed concomitantly with the application of the various abovementioned cytochemical methods, for a morpho-cytochemical analysis.

Periodic Acid-Schiff Method

For the identification of glycogen in blood cells, PAS is the classic method usually recommended (Table 5.1). After blood collection, blood smears are made as usual and air-dried, and the following protocol is recommended:

1. Fix the smear in chilled Gendre's solution for 10 min and allow to air-dry.
2. Wash in running water for 10 min and immerse in 1% periodic acid for 20 min.
3. Wash in running water for 10 min.
4. Treat with Schiff's reagent for 55 min at room temperature.
5. Wash three times in sulfurous water, 3 min each time.
6. Wash in running water for 5 min.
7. Wash quickly in distilled water.
8. Do nuclear staining of the smears with Harris hematoxylin for 3 min, but if the stain is relatively old, the time should be longer.
9. Wash in running water for 10 min.
10. Dehydrate in absolute ethanol: 3 to 5-min baths.
11. Clear in xylene: 3 5-min baths.
12. Mount the slide with Entellan resin.

Carbohydrate energy reserve, specifically glycogen, has been studied by several methods for more than a century. Neukirch in 1910 made the first attempt at a histochemical reaction to demonstrate the presence of glycogen in neutrophils in humans. He found that the granules were soluble in salivary amylase, concluding that these granules in neutrophils represented glycogen (Hayhoe and Quaglino, 1994). Periodic acid oxidizes the hydroxyl radicals of carbohydrates to aldehydes, which react with Schiff's reagent to form a color precipitate. The color produced is classically known as being magenta at sites where glycogen or other carbohydrates of neutral character are found. In the case of blood cells, the positive reaction, with specificity control, indicates the presence of glycogen and can be identified in the cytoplasm of thrombocytes, neutrophils, and eosinophils of fish (Table 5.2 and Fig. 5.1). In the case of PAS-positive granular leukocytes (LG-PAS), the positive reaction even after digestion with salivary amylase indicates the presence of neutral glycoproteins. Hayhoe and Quaglino (1994) cite that in the metachromatic granules of basophils, the positive reaction occasionally observed is due to the presence of phospholipids.

Glycogen is an important energy source for phagocytes (Ueda et al., 2001; Tavares-Dias, 2006b; Shigdar et al., 2009; Zhang et al., 2019), and in mature leukocytes, it makes up cytoplasmic inclusions (Hayhoe and Quaglino, 1994; Lorenzi, 1999), which accumulate during cell maturation (Shigdar et al., 2009). In trout (Oncorhynchus mykiss), during phagocytosis, neutrophils show a PAS-positive reaction (Lamas et al., 1994). The presence of glycogen in phagocytic cells is associated with energy needs to carry out functions.

Phosphatases

In fish and other vertebrates, phosphatases are enzymes distributed in various tissues. Such enzymes constitute a group in which an orthophosphate radical of an organic

Table 5.1. PAS - Periodic acid-Schiff staining (McManus, 1946).

a) Fixer: Gender	b) Sulfurous water
85.0 mL of picric acid saturated in ethanol 96%	10.0 mL of HCl (1 N)
10.0 mL of formol 40%	10.0 mL of sodium bisulfite 10%
5.0 mL of glacial acetic acid	q.s.p. 180.0 mL of distilled water
Keep in refrigerator between 4 and 6°C	Prepare at the time of use
c) Reativo de Schiff	**d) Hematoxilina de Harris**
2.0 g of basic fuchsin	5.0 g of Harris hematoxylin crystals
4.0 g of potassium metabisulfite	50.0 mL of absolute alcohol
2.5 mL of hydrochloric acid	100.0 g of double aluminum and potassium sulfate (potassium alum)
250.0 mL of distilled water	2.5 g of red mercury oxide
6.0 g of activated mineral coal	1000 mL of distilled water
Preparation of the Schiff Reactive	**Preparation of Harris hematoxylin**
a. Heat the water in an oven at 60°C and dilute in fuchsin and metabisulfite.	a. One day before preparing the solution, the hematoxylin must be dissolved in absolute alcohol.
b. After diluting, add hydrochloric acid and mix for one or 2 min.	b. The next day place the potassium alum in distilled and hot water, but without boiling, until it is completely dissolved.
c. Place it in a glass and shake at regular intervals for 30 min.	c. When the potassium alum is dissolved, remove the beaker from the heating plate or fire and add the hematoxylin crystal solution, return to the fire (without boiling), and leave until it reaches a purple color.
d. Add the activated carbon and mix with a glass stick.	d. Remove from the hot plate or fire, and add red mercury oxide. Then, return to heating, leaving steam only.
The solution should be transparent and straw colored and should be stored in amber glass sealed with parafilm, protected with aluminum foil and kept at 4°C. However, the Schiff reagent must be removed from the refrigerator 60 min before use and leave at room temperature.	e. Remove from heating, let it cool; filter and store in amber glass, and always filter after use.
e) Result	**f) Specificity control**
Magenta-colored precipitate in the Periodic acid-Schiff-positive leukocyte cytoplasm and in the form of magenta-colored granules in the thrombocyte cytoplasm.	To control specificity, some blood extensions, after being fixed and washed as described in steps 1-2, are subjected to treatment with salivary amylase (Lison, 1960), in a humid chamber at 37°C for 60 min. Then, the extensions are washed with running water for 10 min, continuing the procedure from steps 2-12 of the method.

phosphate is released. The classification of acid and alkaline phosphatases is based on the optimum pH of the reaction. Its cytochemical demonstration is based on the use of a monobasic sodium salt of alpha-naphthyl phosphate, which after enzymatic hydrolysis leads to the formation of phosphoric acid and alpha-naphthyl, which reacts with a diazonium salt (e.g. fast blue RR) that is placed in the reaction medium to form a stable, colorless, and insoluble final product indicating the site of the enzymatic activity.

Table 5.2. PAS method for glycogen identification in blood cells of 11 freshwater fish species. (Table author's own.)

Species	Thrombocytes	Lymphocytes	Neutrophils	Monocytes	Eosinophils	LG-PAS	Basophils
Oreochromis niloticus	Positive	Negative	Positive	Negative			Positive
Hybrid tilapia	Positive	Negative	Positive	Negative			Negative
Brycon cephalus	Positive	Negative	Positive	Negative			
Brycon orbignyanus	Positive	Negative	Positive	Weak			
Colossoma macropomum	Positive	Negative	Positive	Negative	Weak	Intense	
Piaractus mesopotamicus	Positive	Negative	Positive	Weak	Positive	Intense	
Hybrid "tambacu"	Positive	Negative	Positive	Negative	Weak	Intense	
Leporinus macrocephalus	Weak	Negative	Positive	Negative			Positive
Cyprinus carpio	Positive	Negative	Positive	Negative	Positive	Intense	
Prochilodus lineatus	Positive	Negative	Positive	Negative	Negative		
Ictalurus punctatus	Weak	Negative	Positive	Weak			Negative

LG-PAS = PAS-positive granular leukocyte. Hybrid tilapia: *Oreochromis niloticus* × *Oreochromis aureus*.

Acid phosphatase is an enzyme that characterizes lysosomes and shows high activity in non-specific granules of leukocytes, especially in phagocytes. Its optimal pH is approximately 5.0, and it is directly involved in the process of phagocytosis and responsible for intracellular digestion. In the granulocytes of neutrophils, shortly after the phagocytosis of bacteria or other antigenic substances (Shigdar *et al.*, 2009), the phagosomes fuse with the lysosomes, represented by non-specific granules. Acid phosphatase is inhibited by fluoride ions in the reaction medium (Kiernan, 2008).

Alkaline phosphatase is an enzyme inhibited by iodine, cyanide, and arsenate, and its optimal activity occurs at pH 9.2–9.6 (Jamra and Lorenzi, 1983). This enzyme is present in neutrophil granules only in some species of fish, in neutrophil precursor cells, and in eosinophil and basophil granulocytes where detectable enzyme activity is minimal. In positive neutrophils, this activity is greater in the differentiated cells, therefore in circulating, mature forms. This is true when compared to the young

precursor forms. This indicates that the enzymes reach their highest activity at the end of cell maturation, when cells are then released into circulation by hematopoietic organs.

Method for Alkaline Phosphatase

Alkaline phosphatase activity in fish blood is demonstrated using the method of Ackerman (1962) with modifications (Table 5.3). After blood collection, the following procedure is performed:

1. Prepare blood smears as usual and allow to air-dry.
2. Fix slides in a mixture of absolute methanol-formalin (9:1) at −4°C for 30 s.
3. Wash slides in running water for 10 min and then wash slides rapidly with distilled water and allow to air-dry.
4. Cover smears with incubation medium and incubate for 1-2 h at 37°C.
5. Wash slides under running water for 5 min and then wash rapidly with distilled water.

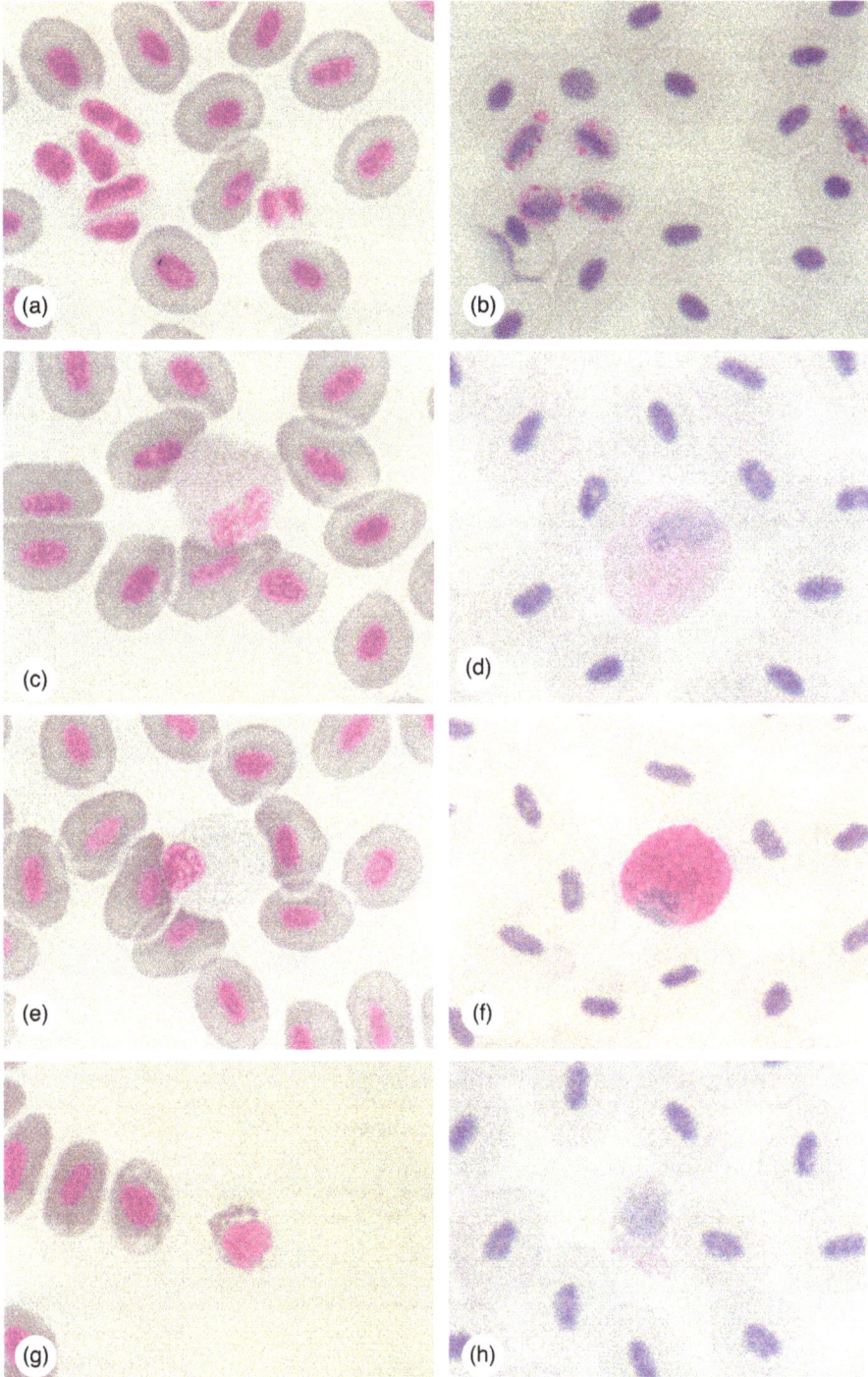

Fig. 5.1. Thrombocytes of pacu, *Piaractus mesopotamicus*, stained with MGGW (a) and PAS (b). Neutrophils of pacu stained with MGGW (c) and PAS (d). LG-PAS of pacu stained with MGGW (e) and PAS (f). Eosinophils of pacu (h). 1000× magnification.

Table 5.3. Alkaline phosphatase method using naphthol AS-MX phosphate. (Table author's own.)

a) Incubation medium	c) Neutral red solution
• 12.0 mg naphthol AS-MX phosphate • 0.2 mL N,N-dimethylformamide • 40.0 mL 0.2 M Tris buffer (pH 9.0)	
Only at the time of staining, dissolve 4 mg of fast blue RR in 4 mL of incubation medium.	• 6 g neutral red • Distilled water: q.s.p. 100 mL
b) 0.2 M Tris-maleate buffer	**d) Control for specificity**
Stock solution Prepare solution A: • 4.7 g Tris (hydroxymethyl) aminomethane. 3.1 g maleic acid in 1000 mL of distilled water.	For control for specificity, do not use naphthol AS-MX phosphate in incubation medium.
Prepare solution B: • 0.2 N NaOH	**e) Result** Blue precipitate in cytoplasm of leukocytes shows positive results for alkaline phosphatase.
Tampon use solution: Add 50.0 mL of solution A to 99.0 mL of solution B and distilled water q.s.p. 200.0 mL.	

6. Do a nuclear staining with 1% neutral red for 6 min and wash rapidly under running water and then with distilled water.

7. Allow to air-dry.

A positive reaction for alkaline phosphatase can be seen in the cytoplasm of neutrophils of different species of fish and sometimes in thrombocytes (Table 5.4 and Fig. 5.2). In *Ictalurus melas*, two phases of maturation of neutrophils were demonstrated: (1) positive for peroxidase (myeloperoxidase) and negative for alkaline phosphatase and (2) positive for alkaline phosphatase and negative or with low activity for peroxidase (myeloperoxidase), indicating that two important maturation phases of neutrophils occur in this species of fish (Garavini *et al.*, 1981), which can be characterized cytochemically.

Method for Acid Phosphatase

For the detection of acid phosphatase in blood cells of fish, the method of Goldberg and Barka (1962) with modifications (Table 5.5) is recommended, according to the following protocol:

1. Fix the blood smears in buffered acetone for 30 s

2. Wash slides under running water for 10 min and then rapidly with distilled water.

3. Cover the smears with incubation and let stand at 37°C for 90 min.

4. Wash under running water for 5 min and then rapidly with distilled water.

5. Stain nuclei with Harris hematoxylin for 3-5 min.

6. Wash under running water and allow to air-dry.

Acid phosphatase hydrolyzes natural or synthetic phosphate esters, releasing orthophosphoric acid in acidic media (pH 4.5–6.0). It is inhibited by fluoride ions at low concentrations. A study of inhibition by tartaric acid should be considered since most acid phosphatase isoenzymes are inhibited by L-tartaric acid. It constitutes an important hydrolase in the attack and killing of phagocytosed microorganisms and acts together with alkaline phosphatase in the primary defense process. Acid phosphatase, a typical enzyme in the lysosome, an organelle responsible for intracellular digestion, is located in the primary or non-specific granules, also known as azurophil granules. Acid phosphatase activity is lower in mature neutrophils compared

Table 5.4. Cytochemical reaction for alkaline phosphatase, by the Naphthol AS-MX phosphate method, in blood cells of 11 species of freshwater fish. (Table author's own.)

Species	Trombócitos	Linfócitos	Neutrófilos	Monócitos	Eosinófilos	LG-PAS	Basófilos
Oreochromis niloticus	Weak	Negative	Negative	Negative	-	-	Negative
Hybrid tilapia	Weak	Negative	Negative	Negative	-	-	Negative
Brycon cephalus	Negative	Negative	Negative	Negative	-	-	-
Brycon orbignyanus	Negative	Negative	Negative	Negative	-	-	-
Colossoma macropomum	Negative	Negative	Positive	Negative	Negative	Negative	-
Piaractus mesopotamicus	Negative	Negative	Positive	Negative	Negative	Negative	-
Hybrid "tambacu"	Negative	Negative	Positive	Negative	Negative	Negative	-
Leporinus macrocephalus	Negative	Negative	Positive	Negative	-	Negative	Negative
Cyprinus carpio	Negative	Negative	Positive	Negative	Negative	Negative	-
Prochilodus lineatus	Positive	Negative	Negative	Negative	Negative	Negative	-
Ictalurus punctatus	Negative	Negative	Negative	Negative	-	Negative	Negative

LG-PAS+ = PAS-positive granular leukocytes. Hibrid tilapia: *Oreochromis niloticus* × *Oreochromis aureus*.

to alkaline phosphatase at this same maturation stage. In agranulocytes, acid phosphatase activity is high in monocytes and low in lymphocytes. Cytochemical electron microscopy shows that T cells exhibit intense positivity in the region of the Golgi apparatus, whereas B cells can be positive or negative. In fish, both lysosomal enzymes are considered important cytochemical markers in the differentiation between neutrophils and eosinophils (Meseguer *et al.*, 1994). Positive staining for acid phosphatase can be found in the cytoplasm of thrombocytes, lymphocytes, monocytes, and neutrophils (Fig. 5.3).

Method for Peroxidase (Myeloperoxidase)

For the detection of myeloperoxidase in blood cells of fish, the ortho-toluidine-hydrogen peroxide method is recommended as described below (Table 5.6).

1. Prepare the blood smears as usual and allow to air-dry.

2. Fix in absolute alcohol-to-formalin (9:1) for 5 min and wash under running water for 10 min.
3. Immerse in incubation medium containing ortho-toluidine-hydrogen peroxide, 15-20 min.
4. Wash under running water for 5 min.
5. Stain nuclei with Harris hematoxylin for 3 min.
6. Wash under running water for 5 min and rapidly with distilled water.
7. Dehydrate in absolute alcohol: three baths of 5 min each.
8. Clear in xylene: three baths of 5 min each.
9. Mount in Entellan.

The purpose of steps 7-9 was to obtain permanent slides.

In fish, a positive reaction to peroxidase can be seen mainly in neutrophils (Fig. 5.4 and Table 5.7). Specific granules of neutrophils are devoid of peroxidase, whereas non-specific or primary granules are positive for peroxidase. As these leukocytes mature, peroxidase activity in their granules increases, making them more evident cytochemically. In the presence

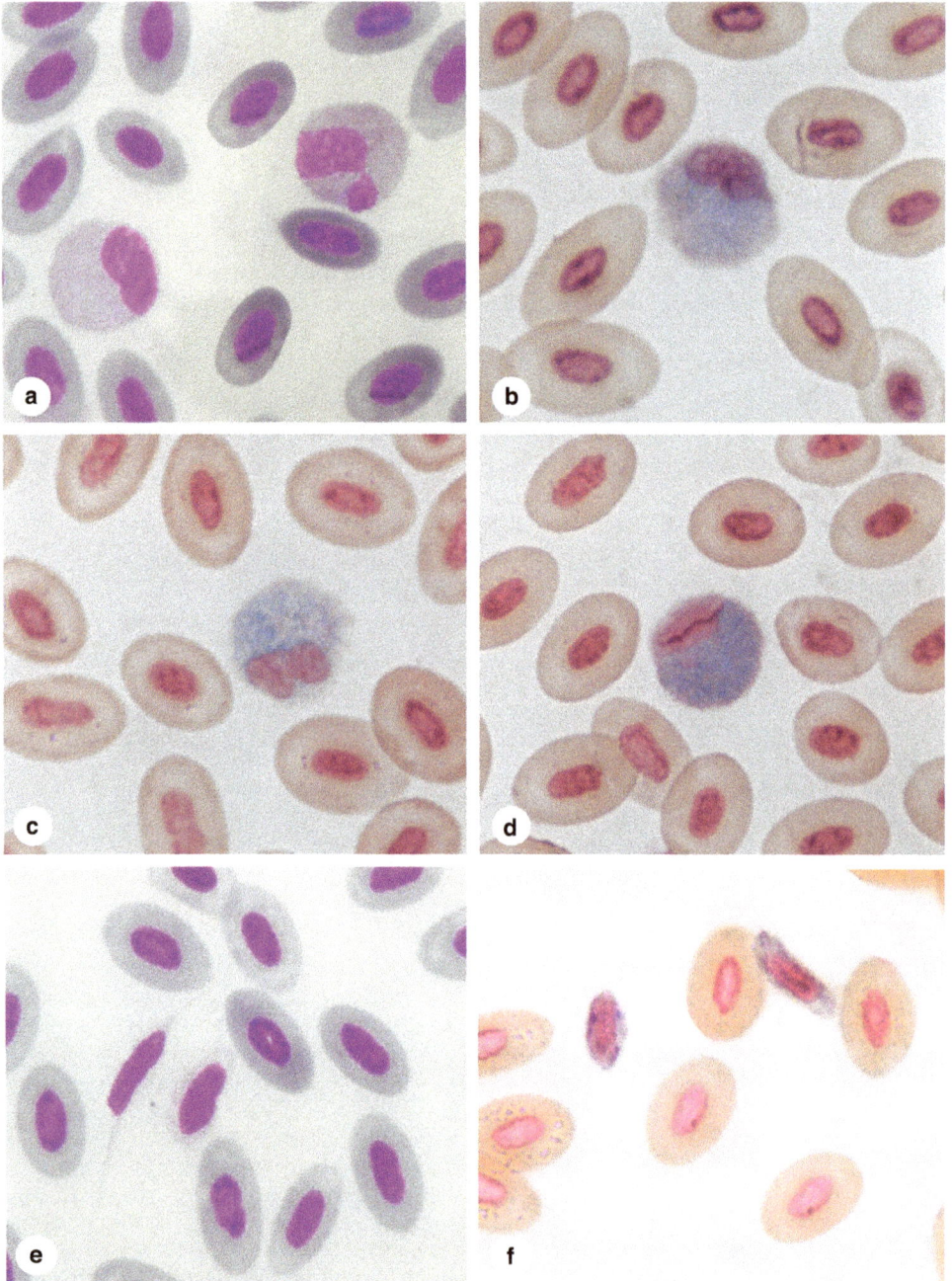

Fig. 5.2. Neutrophils of carp (*Cyprinus carpio*) stained with May-Grünwald-Giemsa (a) and alkaline phosphatase positive (b). Neutrophils of pacu (*Piaractus mesopotamicus*) (c) and tambaqui (*Colossoma macropomum*) (d) alkaline phosphatase positive. Thrombocytes of *Prochilodus lineatus* stained with May-Grünwald-Giemsa (e) and alkaline phosphatase positive (f). 1000× magnification. (Figure author's own.)

Table 5.5. Method for acid phosphatase. (Table author's own).

a) Fixative: buffered acetone	c) Acetate buffer
• 168.0 mL of 0.03 M citric acid	• 14.8 mL of 0.2 M acetic acid
• 32.0 mL of 0.03 M sodium citrate	• 35.2 mL of sodium acetate
• 300.0 mL of acetone	• q.s.p. 100.0 mL of distilled water, pH 5.0
b) Incubation medium	**d) Control for specificity**
a) 7.4 mL of 0.1 M acetate buffer, pH 5.0	
b) 2.0 mg naphthol AS-BI phosphate	
c) 200.0 mL of N,N-dimethylformamide	
d) 160.0 mL 4% pararosaniline in 2 N HCl	Do not use the substrate naphthol AS-BI in the incubation medium.
e) 160.0 mL of 4% sodium nitrite (NaNO2)	
f) 2.6 mL of distilled water	
Mix in this order: first add the items d and e, and then item a, and then add items b and c. Last, add item f, adjusting pH to 4.9-5.0 using 1 M NaOH	**e) Result** Red precipitate in the cytoplasm of positive leukocytes.

of hydrogen peroxide, neutrophil peroxidase catalyzes the oxidation of halide ions, resulting in halogenation of the bacterial cell wall, with its consequent destruction (Azevedo and Lunardi, 2003; Silva *et al.*, 2011). This oxidative lysosomal enzyme modulates phagocytic activity and acts on the intracellular bactericidal system involving oxidation reactions and formation of free radicals (Ueda *et al.*, 2001; Shigdar *et al.*, 2009; Silva *et al.*, 2011). Thus, peroxidase plays an important role in the natural immune response of teleostean fish.

Eosinophilic peroxidase, called EPO, is an enzyme characteristic of secondary or specific granules in eosinophils, which influences two events during the inflammatory process– the marginalization of neutrophils and their involvement at the lesion site. EPO plays an important role in attacking multicellular parasites in higher vertebrates, but in fish this defense role has not been clearly defined, since not all species have circulating eosinophils. In some fish species, the absence of peroxidase appears to be accompanied by the compensatory development of other antibacterial components such as cationic proteins (Fomina *et al.*, 1984; Araújo *et al.*, 2009).

Method for Non-Specific Esterase

Napthyl AS-D acetate is the substrate usually used to demonstrate non-specific esterase, especially in monocytes and their precursors (Table 5.8). After preparing blood smears as usual and air-drying, the following protocol is carried out.

1. Fix blood smears in formalin vapor for 5 min.
2. Wash slides under running water for 5 min.
3. Immerse in recently prepared incubation medium and let it stand at room temperature for 60 min.
4. Wash slides rapidly with distilled water.
5. Stain nuclei with Harris hematoxylin for 3–5 min.
6. Wash smears under running water for 5 min and rinse rapidly with distilled water.
7. Allow stained smears to air-dry.

A positive reaction for non-specific esterase, by the naphthol AS-D acetate esterase method, demonstrated as blue granules of variable intensity, occurs in the cytoplasm of monocytes of various species of fish (Table 5.9 and Fig. 5.5). Esterases are lysosomal enzymes involved in

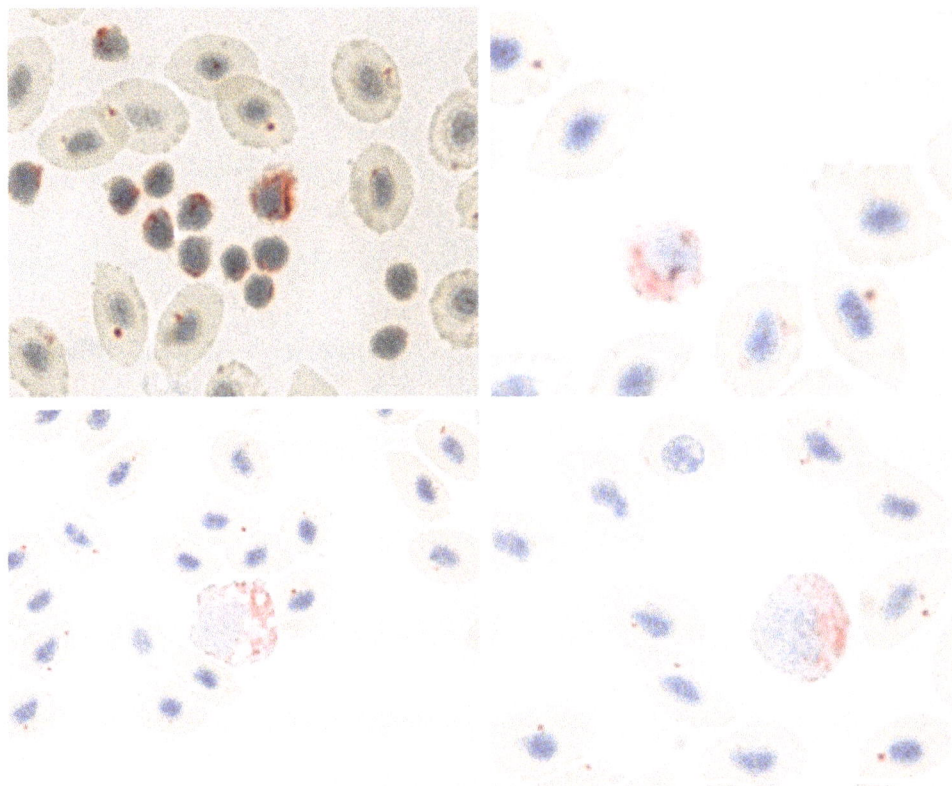

Fig. 5.3. Thrombocytes (a), lymphocytes (b), monocytes (c), and neutrophils (d) of *Centropomus parallelus*, with positive reaction for acid phosphatase. 1280× magnification (Silva *et al.*, 2011).

defense and digestion mechanisms intracellular in phagocytic processes (Tavares-Dias and Barcellos, 2005; Tavares-Dias, 2006b; Silva *et al.*, 2011).

Blue Precipitate in the Cytoplasm of Leukocytes

The esterases constitute a family of enzymes capable of hydrolyzing esters of carboxylic acid and alcohols, phenols, or naphthols. They comprise the carboxyl esterases, aryl esterases, and acetyl esterases. Each of these groups corresponds to a set of enzymes (isoenzymes) closely related to each other. Naphthol esters have been predominantly used in the cytochemistry of esterases, as they allow the formation of a stable, colored final product for analysis under an ordinary light microscope. Doggett *et al.* (1987) demonstrated in fish leukocytes that alpha-naphthyl acetate esterase can be used to distinguish T lymphocytes from B lymphocytes, in which T lymphocytes are positive and B lymphocytes are negative. Alpha-naphthyl acetate esterase and naphthol AS or AS-D acetate are the substrates commonly used for labeling non-specific esterase activity in mononuclear leukocytes (Dacie and Lewis, 1991; Tavares-Dias, 2006a, b). In teleostean fish, naphthol AS-D acetate (NASDA) esterase is a good enzyme for labeling blood monocytes (Tavares-Dias, 2006b). This is an enzyme related to cellular defense mechanisms, facilitation of leukocyte diapedesis, inactivation of toxic products, and destruction of microorganisms (Azevedo and Lunardi, 2003; Silva *et al.*, 2011).

Sudan Black B Method

The classic method of Sudan Black (Table 5.10) is recommended for cytochemical demonstration

Table 5.6. Toluidine-hydrogen peroxide method. (Table author's own.)

a) Incubation medium

- 12.0 mL of absolute alcohol
- 80.0 mL of distilled water
- 0.5 mL of ortho-toluidine
- 1.0 mL of 6% hydrogen peroxide (H2 O2) or 20 volumes.

Ortho-toluidine should be dissolved in absolute alcohol.

b) Control for specificity

Do not include hydrogen peroxide in incubation medium.

c) Result

In the granules of leukocytes, there is a brown precipitate of varied intensity.

of lipids in leukocytes after preparation of the blood smears.

1. Prepare blood smears as usual and allow to air-dry.
2. Fix in 70% ethanol for 5 s (Reingold and Wislocki, 1948).
3. Immerse slides in Sudan Black B for 60 min.
4. Dip slides rapidly in 70% ethanol.
5. Wash under running water for 5 min.
6. Do nuclear staining with Harris hematoxylin for 3 min.
7. Wash slides under running water for 5 min, dip rapidly in distilled water, and allow to air-dry.

Sudan Black B is a liposoluble azo dye; that is, it has the property of being more soluble in non-polar than polar solvents and is therefore able to detect cellular and tissue lipids.

Hematopoietic cells contain finely dispersed lipids in their cytoplasm and complexed structures, such as lipoproteins, which constitute the membrane system of the cell. These lipids cannot be identified in blood smears with any classic hematological stain of the Romanowsky type. Sudan Black B, besides being soluble in lipids, is capable of chemically reacting with unsaturated fatty acids in the cell membrane, conferring a dark color. Leukocyte granulocytes show, in general, Sudan Black B positivity, due to the presence of cytoplasmic granules (Fig. 5.6).

Monocytes display variable positivity, whereas lymphocytes are generally negative. Positivity increases with maturation in the different types of leukocytes.

Thus, immature leukocytes may appear weakly sudanophilic, whereas cells in the final phase of differentiation show strong staining.

Leukocytes contain lipids, which can be detected by Sudan Black B. Neutrophils can use cytoplasmic lipids as an energy source, and, in addition, these cells can degrade lipids through the action of cytoplasmic enzymes (Lorenzi, 1999). Therefore, the sudanophilia in these granulocytes not only reveals the presence of lipids but also provides positivity due to the presence of phospholipids in the membrane made up of unsaturated fatty acids, which chemically react with Sudan Black B. In eosinophils, cytoplasmic granules also show intense sudanophilia (Ueda *et al.*, 2001; Araújo *et al.*, 2009).

Bromophenol Blue Method

There are various methods for demonstrating proteins in general in tissue sections or isolated cells, such as blood cells. One of the most sensitive methods that detects proteins concentrated in cytoplasmic granules in leukocytes is that using mercurial stain bromophenol blue (Waldmann-Meyer and Schilling, 1956). This method allows the demonstration of the presence of this substance in specific granules of eosinophils and neutrophils, for the identification of these granulocytes (Fig. 5.7 and Table 5.11).

For the application of the staining method using the mercurial stain bromophenol blue on blood cells, prepare blood smears as usual, allow to air-dry well, and use the following protocol:

1. Fix blood smears in formol vapor for 10 min.
2. Wash slides under running water for 5 min.
3. Immerse in bromophenol blue solution for 15 min.
4. Dip in 0.5% acetic acid, three times, for 10, 5, and 5 min.
5. Wash in distilled water.
6. Wash in 0.1 M phosphate buffer (pH 7.0) for 3 min.
7. Air-dry.
8. Dip in butanol.
9. Clear as follows:

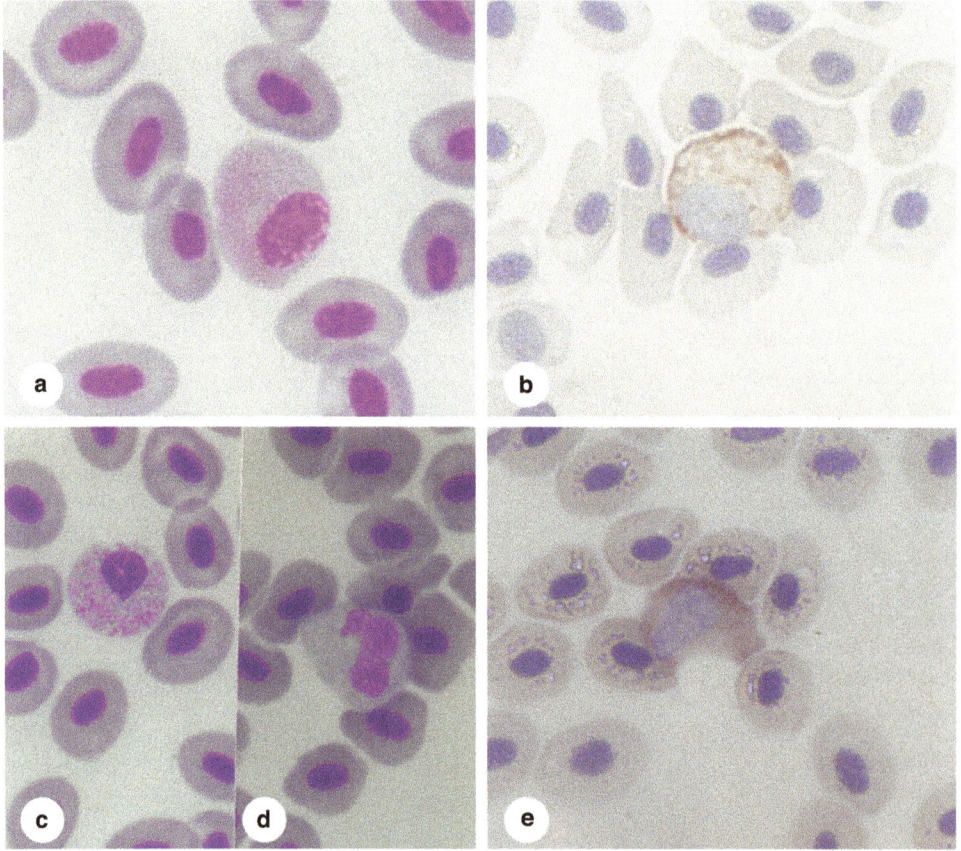

Fig. 5.4. Neutrophils of tambacu hybrid (*Colossoma macropomum* × *Piaractus mesopotamicus*) stained with May-Grünwald-Giemsa-Wright (a) and peroxidase positive (b). Neutrophil (d) and heterophil (c) of matrinxã (*Brycon amazonicus*) stained with May-Grünwald-Giemsa-Wright and peroxidase-positive neutrophil (e). 1000× magnification. (Figure author's own.)

Absolute alcohol + xylene [1:1] – for 3 min; Three baths of xylene, 3 min each; and

10. Mount the slide using Entellan.

Bromophenol blue strongly stains basic proteins present in high concentration in specific granules in eosinophils, which have defense function against microorganisms and parasites, causing their death when they are released by the cells or when they merge with phagosomes.

Metachromatic Staining

The phenomenon of metachromasia is seen when a cationic dye, in process of staining, confers on an anionic substance a different color as the stain itself. This behavior is the result of change in the wavelength when the cationic dye interacts with the anionic sites, for example, of the very negatively charged proteoglycan molecules (Kiernan, 2008). Metachromatic dyes include toluidine blue, methylene blue, thionine, crystal violet, cresyl violet, and safranin. Among these, toluidine is the most used for the demonstrating metachromasia. In the study of blood cells, this method is of great value in identifying the type of granulocyte, namely the basophil (Table 5.12), whose granules contain heparin, a highly negatively charged sulfated glucosamine.

In practice, toluidine blue staining is done according to the following protocol.

Table 5.7. Peroxidase (myeloperoxidase) reaction, by the ortho-toluidine-hydrogen peroxide method, in blood cells of 11 species of freshwater fish. (Table author's own.)

Species	Thrombocytes	Lymphocytes	Neutrophils	Monocytes	Eosinophils	LG-PAS	Basophils
Oreochromis niloticus	Weak	Negative	Positive	Negative	Negative	Negative	Negative
Hybrid tilapia	Negative	Negative	Weak	Weak	-	-	Negative
Brycon cephalus	Weak	Negative	Positive	Negative	-	-	-
Brycon orbignyanus	Negative	Negative	Positive	Negative	-	-	-
Colossoma macropomum	Negative	Negative	Negative	Negative	Negative	Negative	-
Piaractus mesopotamicus	Negative	Negative	Weak	Weak	Negative	Weak	-
Hybrid "tambacu"	Negative	Negative	Weak	Negative	Negative	Weak	-
Leporinus macrocephalus	Negative	Negative	Weak	Weak	-	Weak	Weak
Cyprinus carpio	Negative	Negative	Weak	Negative	Negative	Weak	-
Prochilodus lineatus	Negative	Negative	Negative	Negative	Negative	-	-
Ictalurus punctatus	Weak	Negative	Positive	Weak	-	-	Negative

LG-PAS = PAS-positive granular leukocytes. Hybrid tilapia: *Oreochromis niloticus* × *Oreochromis aureus*.

Table 5.8. Method for non-specific esterase. (Table author's own.)

a) Incubation medium

- 80 mL of 1% propylene glycol in 0.2 M phosphate buffer, pH 6.9
- 0.8 mL of naphthol AS-D acetate 1% diluted in acetone
- 0.16 g of fast blue BB salt

b) Specificity control

For specificity control, do not include naphthol AS-D acetate in the incubation medium and leave some blood extensions in this solution for 60 min and follow steps 4-7

c) Result

Blue-colored precipitate in the leukocyte cytoplasm

Prepare blood smears as usual, allow to air-dry, then fix, and stain the smears as shown below.

1. Fix the blood smears in acetic acid-alcohol (3:1) for 1 min.
2. Wash slides in 70% alcohol for 3 min.
3. Wash in 0.67% citric acid for 35 min.
4. Wash rapidly in distilled water.
5. Immerse in 0.025% toluidine blue for 3 min.
6. Wash rapidly in distilled water and allow to air-dry.

During maturation of the basophils, there is a gradual increase in the size of their granules and also the concentration of heparin within

Table 5.9. Non-specific esterase reaction, by the naphthol AS-D acetate esterase method, in blood cells of 11 species of freshwater fish.

Species	Thrombocytes	Lymphocytes	Neutrophils	Monocytes	Eosinophis	LG-PAS	Basophils
Oreochromis niloticus	Negative	Weak	Negative	Weak	-	-	Negative
Hybrid tilapia	Negative	Weak	Negative	Positive	-	-	Negative
Brycon cephalus	Weak	Weak	Negative	Positive	-	-	-
Brycon orbignyanus	Negative	Weak	Negative	Positive	-	-	-
Colossoma macropomum	Negative	Negative	Negative	Weak	Negative	Negative	-
Piaractus mesopotamicus	Negative	Negative	Negative	Weak	Negative	Negative	-
Hybrid "tambacu"	Negative	Negative	Negative	Weak	Negative	Negative	-
Leporinus macrocephalus	Negative	Weak	Negative	Positive	-	-	Negative
Cyprinus carpio	Weak	Weak	Negative	Weak	Negative	Negative	-
Prochilodus lineatus	Negative	Weak	Negative	Weak	Negative	-	-
Ictalurus punctatus	Weak	Negative	Negative	Positive	-	-	Negative

LG-PAS = PAS-positive granular leukocytes. Hybrid tilapia: *Oreochromis niloticus* × *Oreochromis aureus*

them. When these granules are subjected to the toluidine blue cationic dye method, they appear purple due to the phenomenon of metachromasia (Fig. 5.8). The phenomenon of metachromasia was first described by Ehrlich in 1879 and, as noted earlier, became important because it allows accurate identification of basophils in blood smears.

Among 15 species of fish (*C. macropomum, P. mesopotamicus*, tambacu hybrid, *C. carpio, B. amazonicus, B. orbignyanus, L. macrocephalus, Astronotus ocellatus, Prochilodus lineatus, Hoplias malabaricus, Astyanax bimaculatus, Aristichthys nobilis, O. niloticus*, tilapia hybrid *Oreochromis niloticus* × *Oreochromis aureus*, and *I. punctatus*), only *L. macrocephalus, I. punctatus, O. niloticus*, and tilapia hybrid show basophils in circulating blood (Tavares-Dias, 2006a). Besides that basophils are extremely rare in the circulating blood of fish (Tavares-Dias and Moraes, 2004; Ranzani-Paiva and

Silva-Souza, 2004; Tavares-Dias, 2006b; Pádua and Ishikawa, 2011), sometimes the absence of these granulocytes in blood smears can be due to inadequate application of the classic hematological staining technique. The cytoplasmic granules of basophils are characterized by being water soluble, and mistakes can be made in their preservation. Different protocols for fixing blood smears intended for metachromatic staining have shown that the quality of the reaction can be affected by the use of the fixative and the type of fixative (Tavares-Dias, 2006a). Padua and Ishikawa (2011) demonstrated that the fixation of blood smears with acid-alcohol and under acidic conditions (pH 4.0) results in a metachromatic reaction with excellent quality for identification of blood basophils. In fish, despite the extensive studies on hematology, cytochemistry, and so on, the function of basophils remains unknown.

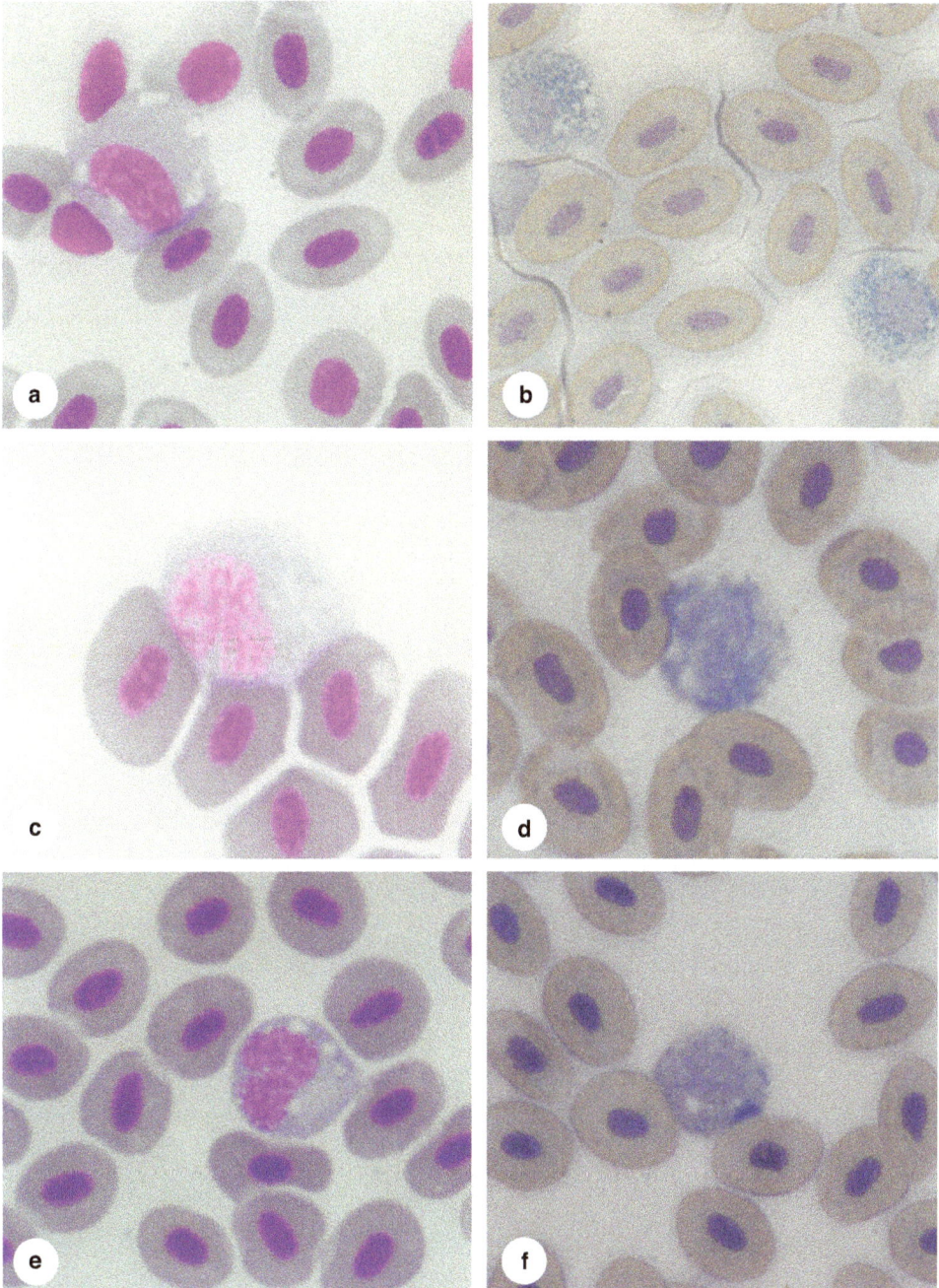

Fig. 5.5. Monocytes of piauçu, *Leporinus macrocephalus*, stained with May-Grünwald-Giemsa (a) and for non-specific esterase (b). Monocytes of red tilapia hybrid (*Oreochromis niloticus* × *Oreochromis aureus*) stained with May-Grünwald-Giemsa (c) and for non-specific esterase (d). Monocytes of matrinxã (*Brycon amazonicus*) stained with May-Grünwald-Giemsa (e) and for non-specific esterase (f). 1000× magnification. (Figure author's own.)

Table 5.10. Sudan Black B method (Lison, 1960).

a) Saturated dye solution

- 0.3 g of Sudan Black B
- 100.0 mL of 70% ethanol

Mix well and let stand.

b) Specificity control

To control specificity, some unstained blood extensions must be subjected to a mixture of chloroform-methanol (1:1), for approximately 1 h at room temperature and follow steps 3-7

c) Result

Sudanophilic cytoplasmic granules in gray tint of varying intensity or black

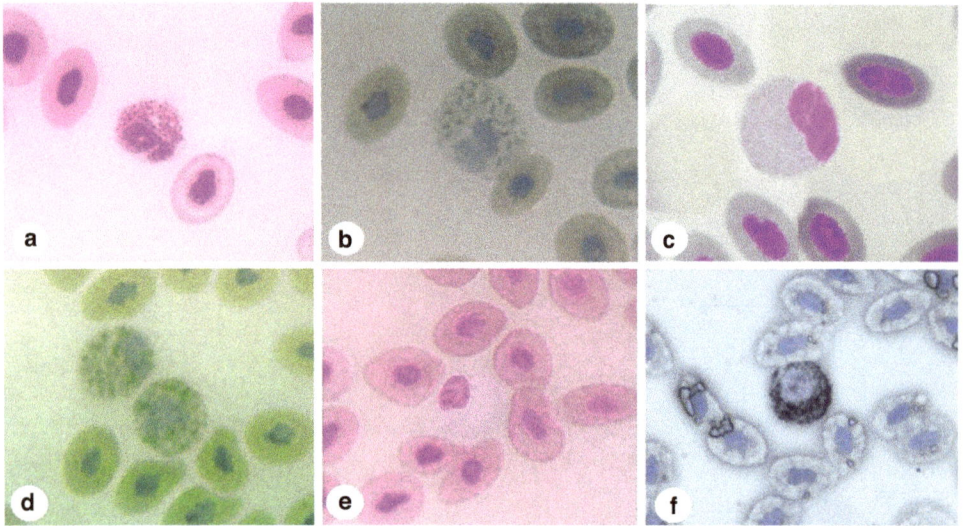

Fig. 5.6. Eosinophils of pirarucu, *Arapaima gigas*, stained with May-Grünwald-Giemsa (a) and Sudan Black-positive granules (b). Neutrophils of pirarucu, *A. gigas*, stained with May-Grünwald-Giemsa (c) and Sudan Black-positive granules (d). 1000× magnification. Neutrophils of fat snook, *Centropomus parallelus*, stained with Leishman's stain (e) and showing positive staining with Sudan Black (f) (Silva *et al.*, 2011). 1280× magnification.

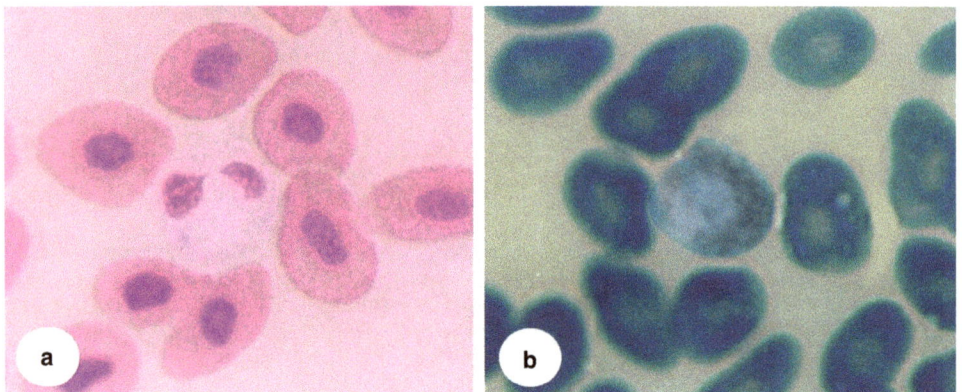

Fig. 5.7. Neutrophils of pirarucu, *Arapaima gigas*, stained with May-Grünwald-Giemsa (a) and bromophenol blue (b). 1000× magnification. (Figure author's own.)

Table 5.11. Bromophenol blue method (Mazia et al., 1953)

a) Staining solution

- 100 mg bromophenol blue
- 10 g mercuric chloride (HgCl2)
- 100 mL of 95% ethanol

b) 0.1 M Sorensen phosphate buffer, pH 7.0

0.2 M phosphate buffer stock solution:

a) 2.78 g monobasic sodium phosphate in 100 mL of distilled water

b) 5.36 g anhydrous dibasic sodium phosphate in 100 mL of distilled water

Preparation of 0.1 M phosphate buffer (pH 7.0)

Add 39.0 mL of solution A (0.2 M) to 61.0 mL of solution B (0.2 M) and add 100 mL of distilled water to obtain 0.1 M buffer.

c) Result

Cytoplasmic granules stained dark blue. Color intensity depends directly on protein concentration.

Table 5.12. Metachromatic staining with toluidine blue (Pádua and Ishikawa, 2011). (Open access.)

a) Acetic acid-alcohol (3.1) fixative

300 mL of absolute ethanol

100 mL of glacial acetic acid

b) Toluidine blue stain (0.025%)

0.25 g toluidine blue

21.01 g citric acid (0.1 M)

28.39 g Na2HPO4 (0.2 M)

Distilled water: q.s.p. 1000 mL

c) Result

Cytoplasmic granules of basophils stain purple.

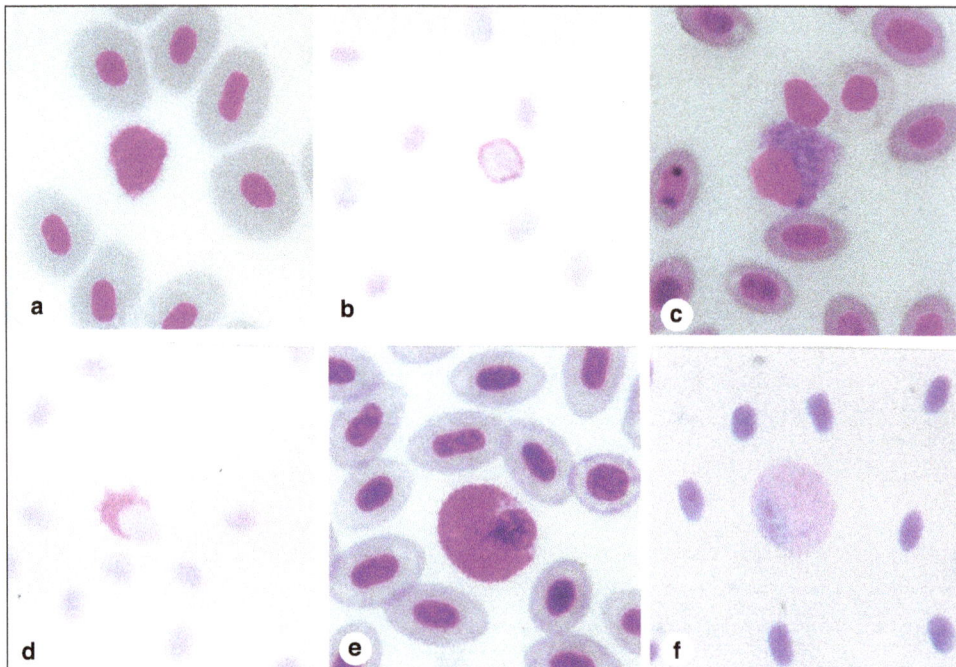

Fig. 5.8. Basophils of catfish, *Ictalurus punctatus*, stained with May-Grünwald-Giemsa (a) and by metachromatic reaction (b). Basophils of Nile tilapia, *Oreochromis niloticus*, stained with May-Grünwald-Giemsa (c) and by metachromatic reaction (d). Basophils of piaugu, *Leporinus macrocephalus*, stained with May-Grünwald-Giemsa (e) and by metachromatic reaction (f). 1000× magnification (Tavares-Dias, 2006a).

References

Ackerman, G.A. (1962) Substituted naphthol As-phosphate derivatives for the localization of leukocyte alkaline phosphatase activity. *Laboratory Investigation* 11, 563–567.

Adhikari, S., Sarkar, B., Chatterjee, A., Mahapatra, C.T. and Ayyappan, S. (2004) Effects of cypermethrin and carbofuran on certain hematological parameters and prediction of their recovery in a freshwater teleost, *Labeo rohita* (Hamilton). *Ecotoxicology and Environmental Safety* 58, 220–226.

Affonso, E.G., Silva, E.C., Tavares-Dias, M., Menezes, G.C., Carvalho, C.S.M. *et al.* (2007) Effect of high levels of dietary vitamin C on the blood responses of matrinxã (*Brycon amazonicus*). *Comparative Biochemistry and Physiology: Part A* 147, 383–388.

Andrade, J.I.A., Ono, E.A., Menezes, G.C., Martins-Brasil, E., Roubach, R. *et al.* (2007) Influence of diets supplemented with vitamins C and E on pirarucu (*Arapaima gigas*) blood parameters. *Comparative Biochemistry and Physiology: Part A* 146, 576–580.

Aragort, W., Alvarez, M.F., Leiro, J.L. and Sanmartín, M.L. (2005) Blood protozoans in elasmobranchs of the family Rajidae from Galicia (NW Spain). *Diseases of Aquatic Organisms* 65, 63–68.

Araújo, C.S.O., Tavares-Dias, M., Gomes, A.L.S., Andrade, S.M.S., Lemos, J.R.G. *et al.* (2009) Infecções parasitárias e parâmetros sanguíneos em *Arapaima gigas* Schinz, 1822 (Arapaimidae) cultivados no estado do Amazonas, Brasil. In: Tavares-Dias, M. (Org). *Manejo e Sanidade de peixes em cultivo*. Embrapa Amapá, Macapá, Brazil, pp. 389–424.

Azevedo, A. and Lunardi, L.O. (2003) Cytochemical characterization of eosinophlic leukocytes circulanting in the blood de turtle (*Chrysemys dorbignih*). *Acta Histochemical* 105, 99–105.

Barber, D.L. and Westermann, J.E.M. (1975) Morphological and histological studies on a P.A.S. positive granular leucocyte in blood and connective tissue of *Catostomus commerssoni* Lacépède (Teleostei:Pisces). *American Journal of Anatomy* 142, 205–220.

Barcelos, L.J.G., Kreutz, L.C., Souza, C., Rodrigues, L.B., Fioreze, I. *et al.* (2004) Hematological changes in jundiá (*Rhamdia quelen* Quoy and Gaimard Pimelodidae) after acute and chronic stress caused by usual aquacultural management, with enfasis on immunosupressive effect. *Aquaculture* 237, 229–236.

Barros, M.M., Pezzato, L.E., Kleemann, G.K., Hisano, H. and Rosa, G.J.M. (2002) Níveis de Vitamina C e Ferro para tilápia do Nilo (*Oreochromis niloticus*). *Revista Brasileira de Zootecnia* 31(6), 2149–2156.

Barros, M.M., Ranzani-Paiva, M.J.T., Pezzato, L.E., Falcon, D.R. and Guimarães, I.G. (2009) Hematological response and growth performance of Nile tilapia fed diets containing folic acid. *Aquaculture Research* 40, 895–903.

Belo, M.A.A., Schalck, S.H.C., Moraes, F.R., Solaris, V.E., Otoboni, A.M.M.B. and Moraes, J.E.R. (2005) Effect of dietary supplementation with vitamin E and stocking density on macrophage recruitment and giant cell formation in the teleost fish, *Piaractus mesopotamicus*. *Journal of Comparative Pathology* 133, 146–154.

Biller, J.D. and Chagas, E. (2022) Mechanisms of resistance and tolerance against parasites in fish: The impairments caused by *Neoechinorhynchus buttnerae* in *Colossoma macropomum*. *Anais da Academia Brasileira de Ciências* 94(4), e20210258.

Biller, J.D. and Takahashi, L.S. (2018) Oxidative stress and fish immune system: Phagocytosis and leukocyte respiratory burst activity. *Anais da Academia Brasileira de Ciências* 90(7). doi:10.1590/0001-3765201820170730.

Blaxhall, P.C. and Daisley, K.W. (1973) Routine haematological methods for use with fish blood. *Journal of Fish Biology* 5(6), 771–781.

Bolasina, S.N. (2006) Cortisol and hematological response in Brazilian codling, *Urophycis brasiliensis* (Pisces, Phycidae) subjected to anesthetic treatment. *Aquaculture International* 14(6), 569–575.

Borges, A., Scotti, L.V., Siqueira, D.R., Zanini, R., Amaral, F., Jurinitz, D.F. and Wassermann, G.F. (2007) Changes in hematological and serum biochemical values in Jundiá *Rhamdia quelen* due to sublethal toxicity of cypermethrin. *Chemosphere* 69, 920–926.

Clauss, T.M., Dove, A.D.N. and Arnold, J.E. (2008) Hematologic disorders of fish. *Veterinary Clinics Exotics Animal Practice* 11, 445–462.

Claver, J.A. and Quaglia, A.I.E. (2009) Comparative morphology, development, and function of blood cells in nonmamalian vertebrates. *Journal of Exotic Pet Medicine* 18(2), 87–97.

Collier, H.B. (1944) The standardizations of blood haemoglobin determinations. *Canadian Medical Association Journal* 50, 550–552.

Crestani, M., Menezes, C., Glusczak, L., Miron, D.S., Lazari, R. *et al.*. (2006) Effects of clomazone herbicide on hematological and some parameters of protein and carbohydrate metabolism of silver catfish *Rhamdia quelen*. *Ecotoxicology and Environmental Safety* 65, 48–55.

Cunha, D.M., Calixto, F.A.A., Takata, R., Portugal, A.C.B., Uehara, S.A., Martins, G.R.F.C., Fonseca, A.B.M., Mesquita, E.F.M. and Almosny, N.R.P. (2021) Morphological and cytochemical characterization of the peripheral blood cells of farmed streaked prochilod Prochilodus lineatus (Characiformes, Prochilodontidae). *Arquivo Brasileiro de Medicina Veterinária e Zootecnia* 73(6), 1312–1333.

Dacie, J.V. and Lewis, S.M. (1991) *Practical Haematology*. Churchill Livingstone, London.

Das, B.K. and Mukherjee, S.C. (2003) Toxicity of cypermethrin in *Labeo rohita* fingerlings: Biochemical, enzymatic and haematological consequences. *Comparative Biochemistry and Physiology: Part C* 134, 109–121.

Davies, A.J., Reed, C.C. and Smit, N.J. (2003) An unusual intraerythrocytic parasite of *Parablennius cornutus* from South Africa. *Journal of Parasitology* 89(5), 913–917.

Delbon, M.C. (2006) *Ação da benzocaína e do óleo de cravo sobre parâmetros fisiológicos de tilápia, Oreochromis niloticus*. Dissertação (Mestrado em Aquicultura), Centro de Aquicultura da Unesp, Jaboticabal, Brazil, 91 pp.

Delbon, M.C. (2010) *Análises cromatográficas e parâmetros hematológicos de tilápia, Oreochromis niloticus, anestesiadas com eugenol em condições laboratoriais e de transporte*. Tese (Doutorado em Aquicultura), Centro de Aquicultura da Unesp, Jaboticabal, Brazil, 115 pp.

Diniz, J.A., Silva, E.O., Souza, W. and Lainson, R. (2002) Some observations on the fine structure of trophozoites of the haemogregarine *Cyrilia lignieresi* (Adeleina: Haemogregarinidae) in erythrocytes of the fish *Synbranchus marmoratus* (Synbranchidae). *Parasitology Research* 88, 593–597.

Doggett, T.A., Wrathmell, A.B. and Harris, J.E. (1987) A cytochemical and ligth microscopical study of the peripheral blood leucocytes of *Oreochromis mossambicus*, Cichlidae. *Journal of Fish Biology* 31, 147–153.

Eiras, J.C., Takemoto, R.M. and Pavanelli, G.C. (2000) *Métodos de estudo e técnicas laboratoriais em parasitologia de peixes*. Vol. 500. EDUEM, Maringá, Brazil. 171 pp.

El-Sayed, Y.S., Saad, T.T. and El-Bahr, S.M. (2007) Acute intoxication of deltamethrin in monosex Nile tilapia, *Oreochromis niloticus* with special reference to the clinical, biochemical and haematological effects. *Environmental Toxicology and Pharmacology* 24, 212–217.

Ferrari, J.E.C., Barros, M.M., Pezzato, L.E., Golçalves, G.S., Hisano, H. and Kleemann, G.K. (2004) Níveis de cobre em dietas para a tilápia do Nilo, *Oreochromis niloticus*. *Acta Scientiarum: Animal Science* 26(4), 429–436.

Gabriel, U.U., Ezeri, G.M.O. and Opabunmi, O.O. (2004) Influence of sex, source, health status and acclimatation on the haematology of *Clarias gariepinus* (Burch, 1822). *African Journal of Biotechnology* 3(9), 463–467.

Garavini, C., Martelli, P. and Borelli, B. (1981) Alkaline pH and peroxidase in neutrophils of the catfish *Ictalurus melas* (Rafinesque) (Siluriformes: Ictaluridae). *Histochemistry* 72, 75–81.

Garcia, F. and Moraes, F.R. (2009) Hematologia e sinais clínicos de *Piaractus mesopotamicus* infectados experimentalmente com *Aeromonas hydrophila*. *Acta Scientiarum: Biological Science* 31(1), 17–21.

Ghiraldelli, L., Martins, L.M., Yamashita, M.M. and Jeronimo, G.T. (2006) Ectoparasites influence on the haematological parameters of Nile tilapia and carp culture in the state of Santa Catarina South Brazil. *Journal of Fisheries and Aquatic Science* 1, 270–276.

Goldberg, A.F. and Barka, T. (1962) Acid phosphatase activity in human blood cells. *Nature* 195:297.

Goldenfarb, P.B., Bowyer, F.P., Hall, E. and Brosious, E. (1971) Reproducibility in the hematology laboratory: The microhematocrit determinations. *American Journal of Clinical Pathology* 56(1), 35–39.

Haddad V., Jr., Garrone Neto, D., Paula Neto, J.B., Marques, F.P.L. and Barbaro, K.C. (2004) Freshwater: Study of epidemiologic, clinic and therapeutic aspects based on 84 envenomings in humans and some enzymatic activities of the venom. *Toxicon* 43, 287–294.

Harr, K.E., Raskin, R.E. and Heard, D.J. (2005) Temporal effects of 3 commonly used anticoagulants on hematologic and biochemical variables in blood samples from Macaws and Burmese pythons. *Veterinary Clinical Pathology* 34(4), 383–388.

Hassan A.A., Akinsanya B. and Adegbaju W.A. (2007) Haemoparasites of *Clarias gariepinus* and *Synodontis clarias* from Lekki Lagoon, Lagos Nigeria. *Journal of American Science* 3(3), 61–67.

Hattingh, J. (1975) Heparin and ethylenediamine tetra-acetate as anticoagulants for fish blood. *Pflugers Archive European Journal of Physiology* 355(4), 347–352.

Hayhoe, F.G.J. and Quaglino, D. (1994) *Haematological Cytochemistry*. Churchill Livingstone, London.

Hisano, H., Barros, M.M. and Pezzato, L.E. (2007) Levedura e zinco como pró-nutrientes para tilápia-do-nilo (*Oreochromis niloticus*): Aspectos hematológicos. *Boletim do Instituto de Pesca* 33(1), 35–42.

Hrubec, T.C. and Smith, S.A. (1998) Hematology of fishes. In: Feldman, B.F., Zinkl, J.G. and Jain, M.C. (eds) *Schalm's Veterinary Hematology*, 5th edn. Wiley-Blackwell, Blackburg, Virginia, pp. 1120–1125.

Hrubec, T.C. and Smith, S.A. (2010) Hematology of fishes. In: Weiss, D.J. and Wardrop, K.J. (eds) *Schalm's Veterinary Hematology*, 6th edn. Wiley-Blackwell, Ames, Iowa, pp. 994–1003.

Hrubec, T.C., Smith, S.A. and Robertson, J.L. (2001) Age-related changes in hematology and plasma chemistry values of hybrid striped bass (*Morone chrisops* x *Morone saxatilis*). *Veterinary Clinical Pathology* 30(1), 8–15.

Inoue, L.A.K.A., Boijink, C.L., Ribeiro, C.L., Silva, A.M.D. and Affonso, E.G. (2011) Avaliação de respostas metabólicas do tambaqui exposto ao eugenol em banhos anestésicos. *Acta Amazonica* 41(2), 327–332.

Inoue, L.A.K.A., Hackbarth, A. and Moraes, G. (2004) Avaliação dos anestésicos 2-phenoxyethanol e benzocaína no manejo do matrinxã *Brycon cephalus* (Günther, 1869). *Biodiversidade Pampeana* 2, 10–15.

Ishikawa, N.M., Ranzani-Paiva, M.J.T. and Lombardi, J.V. (2008) Total leukocyte counts methods in fish, *Oreochromis niloticus*. *Archives of Veterinary Science* 13(1), 54–63.

Ishikawa, M.M., Pádua, S.B., Satake, F., Hisano, H., Jerônimo, G.T. and Martins, M.L. (2010) Heparina e Na EDTA como anticoagulantes para surubim híbrido (*Pseudoplatystoma reticulatum* x *P. corruscans*): Eficácia e alterações hematológicas. *Ciência Rural* 40(7), 1557–1561.

Ishikawa, M.M., Pádua, S.B., Satake, F., Martins, M.L. and Tavares Dias, M. (2011) Identificação morfológica de organismos semelhantes à Anaplasmataceae em monócitos de surubim híbrido *(Pseudoplatystoma reticulatum* x *P. corruscans)*: Relato de caso. *Revista Brasileira de Medicina Veterinária* 33(4). http://www.alice.cnptia.embrapa.br/alice/handle/doc/917151

Jamra, M. and Lorenzi, T.F. (1983) *Leucócitos, leucemias e linfomas*. Guanabara Koogan, Rio de Janeiro, Brazil.

Jannini, P. and Jannini Filho, P. (1995) *Interpretação clínica do hemograma*, 9ª edn. Savier., São Paulo, Brazil, 625 pp.

Jensch, B.E., Jr. (2002) *Atividade fagocítica do macrófago do curimbatá Prochilodus scrofa (Steindachner 1881)*. Dissertação (Mestrado em Ciências—Biologia Celular e Tecidual). Universidade de São Paulo, São Paulo, Brazil, 80 pp.

Jerônimo, G.T., Laffitte, L.V., Speck, G.M. and Martins, M.L. (2011) Seasonal influence on the hematological parameters in cultured Nile tilapia from southern Brazil. *Brazilian Journal of Biology* 71(3), 719–725.

Kiernan, J.A. (2008) *Histological and Histochemical Methods: Theory and Practice*. Scion, Bloxham, UK.

Kirschbaum, A.A., Seriani, R., Pereira, C.D.S., Assunção, A., Abessa, D.M.S., Rotundo, M.M. and Ranzani-Paiva, M.J.T. (2009) Cytogenotoxicity biomarkers in fat snook, *Centropomus parallelus*, from Cananéia and São Vicente estuaries, SP, Brazil. *Genetics and Molecular Biology* 32(1), 151–154.

Lainson, R. (2007) *Theileria electrophorin*.sp., a parasite of the electric eel *Electrophorus electricus* (Osteichthyes: Cypriniformes: Gymnotidae) from Amazonian Brazil. *Memórias do Instituto Oswaldo Cruz* 102(2), 155–157.

Lamas, J., Santos, Y., Bruno, D.W., Toranzo,A.E. and Anadón, R. (1994) Non-specific cellular responses of rainbow trout to *Vibrio anguillarum* and its e intracellular products (ECPs). *Journal of Fish Biology* 45, 839–854.

Lison, L. (1960) Lipides et lipoproteines. In: Lison, L. (ed.) *Histochimie et cytochimie animales*. Principes et méthodes. Vol. 2. Gauthier Villares, Paris, France, pp. 449–530.

Lorenzi, T.F. (1999) *Manual de hematologia propedêutica e clínica*. MDSI, São Paulo, Brazil.

Maciel, P.O., Affonso, E.G., Boijink, C.L., Tavares-Dias, M. and Inoue, L.A.K.A. (2011) *Myxobolus* sp. (Myxozoa) in the circulating blood of *Colossoma macropomum* (Osteichthyes, Characidae). *Revista Brasileira de Parasitologia Veterinária* 20(1), 82–84.

Martins, M.L., Tavares-Dias, M., Fujimoto, R.Y., Onaka, E.M. and Nomura, D.T. (2004) Haematological alterations of *Leporinus macrocephalus* (Osteichtyes: Anostomidae) naturally infected by *Goezia leporini* (Nematoda: Anisakidae) in fish pond. *Arquivo Brasileiro de Medicina Veterinária e Zootecnia* 56(5), 640–646.

Martins, M.L., Mouriño, J.L.P., Amaral, G.V., Vieira, F.N., Dotta, G. *et al*. (2008a) Haematological changes in Nile tilápia experimentally infected with *Enterococcus* sp. *Brazilian Journal of Biology* 68(3), 631–637.

Martins, M.L., Vieira, F.N., Jerônimo, G.T., Mouriño, J.L.P., Dotta, G. *et al*. (2008b) Leukocyte response and phagocytic activity in Nile tilápia experimentally infected with *Enterococcus* sp. *Fish Physiology and Biochemical* 68:635.

Martins, M.L., Myiazaki, D.M.Y., Tavares-Dias, M., Fenerick, J., Jr., Onaka, E.M. *et al*. (2009) Caracterization of the acute inflammatory response in the hybrid tambacu (*Piaractus mesopotamicus* male x *Colossoma macropomum* female) (Osteichthyes). *Brazilian Journal of Biology* 69(2), 631–637.

Matos, M.S. and Matos, P.F. (1995) *Laboratório clinico médico veterinário*, 2a edn. Atheneu, São Paulo, Brazil.

Matushima, E.R. and Mariano, M. (1996) Kinects of the inflammatory reaction induced by carrageenin in the swinbladder of *Oreochromis niloticus* (Nile tilapia). *Brazilian Journal of Veterinary Research and Animal Science* 33(1), 5–10.

Mazia, D., Brewer, P.A. and Alfert, M. (1953) The cytochemical staining and measurement of protein with mercuric bromophenol blue. *Biological Bulletin* 104, 57–67.

McManus, J.F.A. (1946) Histological demonstration of mucin after periodic acid. *Nature* 158:202.

Melo, J.F.B., Tavares-Dias, M., Lundestedt L.M. and Moraes, G. (2006) Efeito do conteúdo de proteína na dieta sobre os parâmetros hematológicos e metabólicos do bagre sul americano *Rhamdia quelen*. *Revista Ciência Agroambiental* 1(1), 43–51.

Menezes, R.C., Santos, S.M.C., Ceccarelli, P.S., Tavares, L.E.R., Tortelly, R. and Luque, J.L. (2011) Tissue alterations in pirarucu, *Arapaima gigas,* infected by *Goezia spinulosa* (Nematoda). *Revista Brasileira de Parasitologia Veterinária* 20(2), 207–209.

Meseguer, J., López-Ruiz, A. and Angeles-Esteban, M. (1994) Cytochemical characterization of leucocytes from the seawater teleost, gilthead seabream (*Sparus aurata* L.). *Histochemistry* 102, 37–44.

Nakamoto, W., Silva, A.J., Machado, P.E.A. and Padovani, C.R. (1991) Glóbulos brancos e *Cyrilia gomesi* (hemoparasita) em *Synbranchus marmoratus* Bloch, 1795. (Pisces, Synbranchidae) da região de Birigui, SP. *Revista Brasileira de Biologia* 51(4), 755–761.

Napoleão, S.R. (2007) *Análises hematológicas, bioquímicas e hormonais de tubarão-lixa, Ginglymostoma cirratum (Bonnaterre, 1788), em cativeiro, no Brasil*. Dissertação (Mestra em Aquicultura e Pesca)-Instituto de Pesca, São Paulo, Brazil, 47 pp.

Natt, M.P. and Herrick, C.A. (1952) A new blood diluents for counting the erythrocytes and leucocytes of the chicken. *Poultry Science* 31(4), 735–738.

Orecka-Grabda, T. and Wierzbicka, J. (1998) Development of hemogregarines (Apicomplexa), blood parasites of eel, *Anguilla anguilla* (L.). *Acta Ichthyologica et Piscatoria* 28(2), 63–68.

Pádua, S.B. and Ishikawa, M.M. (2011) Metacromasia para identificação de basófilos sanguíneos em surubim híbrido: Contribuição metodológica. *Revista Brasileira de Medicina Veterinária* 33, 147–150.

Pádua, S.B., Ishikawa, M.M., Satake, F., Hisano, H. and Tavares Dias, M. (2009) Valores para o leucograma e trombograma de juvenis de dourado (*Salminus brasiliensis*) em condições experimentais de cultivo. *Revista Brasileira de Medicina Veterinária* 31(4), 282–287.

Pádua, S.B., Ventura, A.S., Satake, F. and Ishikawa, M.M. (2010) Características morfológicas, morfométricas e citoquímicas das células sanguíneas da arraia ocelada *Potamotrygon motoro* (Elasmobranchii, Potamotrygonidae): Estudo de caso. *Ensaios de Ciência* 14(1), 147–158.

Pádua, S.B., Ishikawa, M.M., Satake, F., Jerônimo, G.T. and Pilarski, F. (2011) First record of *Trypanosoma* sp. (Protozoa: Kinetoplastida) in tuvira (*Gymnotus* aff. *inaequilabiatus*) in the Pantanal wetland, Mato Grosso do Sul State, Brazil. *Revista Brasileira de Parasitologia Veterinária* 20(1), 85–87.

Pádua, S.B., Pilarski, F., Sakabe, R., Dias-Neto, J., Chagas, E.C. and Ishikawa, M.M. (2012) Heparina e K3 EDTA como anticoagulantes para tambaqui (Colossoma macropomum Cuvier, 1816). *Acta Amazonica* 42, 293–298.

Pazooki, J. and Masoumian, M. (2004) *Cryptobia acipenseris* and *Haemogregarina acipenseris* infections in *Acipenser guldenstadti* and *A. persicus* in the Southern part of the Caspian Sea. *Journal of Agriculture Science and Technology* 6, 95–101.

Petric, M.C. (2000) *Efeito da suplementação alimentar com vitamina C sobre a formação de gigantócitos em lamínulas de vidro implantadas em tecido subcutâneo de pacus (Piaractus mesopotamicus Holmberg, 1887)*. Dissertação de Mestrado—Medicina Veterinária. UNESP Jaboticabal, Jaboticabal, Brazil, 86 pp.

Pitombeira, M.S. and Martins, J.M. (1966) A direct method for white blood cell count in fishes. *Arquivos da Estação de Biologia Marinha da Universidade Federal do Ceará* 6(2): 605.

Ranzani-Paiva, M.J.T. (1995a) Características hematológicas de tainha, *Mugil platanus* Günther, 1880 (Osteichthyes, Mugilidae) da região estuarino-lagunar de Cananéia—SP (Lat. 25° 00′S—Long. 47° 55′W). *Boletim do Instituto de Pesca* 22(1), 1–22.

Ranzani-Paiva, M.J.T. (1995b) Células sangüíneas e contagem diferencial dos leucócitos de tainha, *Mugil platanus* Günther, 1880 (Osteichthyes, Mugilidae) da região estuarino-lagunar de Cananéia—SP (Lat. 25° 00′S—Long. 47° 55′W). *Boletim do Instituto de Pesca* 22(1), 23–40.

Ranzani-Paiva, M.J.T. (1996) Células sangüíneas e contagem diferencial dos leucócitos em pirapitinga do sul, *Brycon* sp., sob condições experimentais de criação intensiva. *Revista Ceres* 43(250), 685–696.

Ranzani-Paiva, M.J.T. (2007) Hematologia como ferramenta para a avaliação da saúde de peixes. In: Barros, M.M. and Pezzato, L.E. (eds) *2°. Simpósio de Nutrição e Saúde de Peixes, Anais*. . . . . Universidade Estadual Paulista, Botucatu, Brazil, pp. 47–51.

Ranzani-Paiva, M.J.T. and Godinho, H.M. (1983) Sobre células sangüíneas e contagem diferencial de leucócitos e eritroblastos em curimbatá, *Prochilodus scrofa*, Steindachner, 1881(Osteichthyes, Cypriniformes, Prochilodontidae). *Revista Brasileira de Biologia* 43(4), 331–338.

Ranzani-Paiva, M.J.T. and Silva-Solza A.T. (2004) Hematologia de Peixes Brasileiros. In: Ranzani-Paiva, M.J.T., Takemoto, R.M. and Lizama, M.A.P. (Org) *Sanidade de Organismos Aquáticos*. Vol. 1. Livraria Varela, São Paulo, Brazil, pp. 89–120.

Ranzani-Paiva, M.J.T., Ishikawa, C.M., Campos, B.E.S. and Eiras, A.C. (1997) Hematological characteristics associated with parasitism in mullets, *Mugil platanus* Günther, from the estuarine region of Cananéia, São Paulo, Brazil. *Revista brasileira de Zoologia* 14(2), 329–339.

Ranzani-Paiva, M.J.T., Tabata, Y.A. and das Eiras, A.C. (1998) Hematologia comparada entre diplóides e triplóides de truta arco-íris, *Oncorhynchus mykiss* Walbaum (Pisces, Salmonidae). *Revista brasileira de Zoologia* 15(4), 1093–1102.

Ranzani-Paiva, M.J.T., Ishikawa, C.M., Eiras, A.C. and Silveira, V.R. (2004) Effects of an experimental challenge with *Mycobacterium marinum* on the blood parameters of Nile tilapia, *Oreochromis niloticus* (Linnaeus, 1757). *Brazilian Archives of Biology and Technology* 47(6), 945–953.

Ranzani-Paiva, M.J.T., Felizardo, N.N. and Luque, J.L. (2005) Parasitological and hematological analysis of Nile tilapia, *Oreochromis niloticus* Linnaeus, 1757, from Guarapiranga Reservoir, São Paulo State, Brazil. *Acta Scientiarum, Biological Science* 27(3), 231–237.

Reingold, J.J. and Wislocki, G.B. (1948) Histochemical methods applied to haematology. *Blood* 3, 641–655.

Ribeiro, R.D., Ranzani-Paiva, M.J.T., Ishikawa, C.M., Lopes, R.A., Albuquerquer, S. and Carraro, A.A. (1996) Tripanossomos de peixes brasileiros. XVI. *Tryposoma platanusi* sp.n. encontrado na tainha, *Mugil platanus* Günther, 1980 (Pisces, Mugilidae) capturada na região estuarino-lagunar de Cananéia, Estado de São Paulo, Brasil. *Revista Brasileira de Biologia* 56(2), 263–267.

Ribeiro, W.R. (1978) *Contribuição ao estudo de hematologia de peixes. Morfologia e citoquímica das células do sangue e dos tecidos hematopoéticos do mandi amarelo, Pimelodus maculatos Lacépède, 1803*. Tese de Doutorado, Universidade de São Paulo, Ribeirão Preto, Brazil, 110 pp.

Rosenfeld, G. (1947) Corante pancrômico para hematologia e citologia clínica. Nova combinação dos componentes do May-Grünwald e do Giemsa num só corante de emprego rápido. *Memórias do Instituto Butantan* 20, 329–334.

Santos, A.A., Egami, M.I., Ranzani-Paiva, M.J.T. and Juliano, Y. (2009) Hematological parameters and phagocytic activity in fat snook (*Centropomus parallelus*): Seasonal variation, sex and gonadal maturation. *Aquaculture* 296(3–4), 359–366.

Satake, F., Pádua, S.B. and Ishikawa, M.M. (2009) Distúrbios morfológicos em células sanguíneas de peixes em cultivo: uma ferramenta prognóstica. In: Tavares-Dias, M. (ed.) *Manejo e sanidade de peixes em cultivo.* Embrapa Amapá, Macapá, Brazil, pp. 330–345.

Seriani, R. and Ranzani-Paiva, M.J.T. (2012) Alterações hematológicas em peixes: Aspectos fisiopatológicos e aplicações em ecotoxicologia aquático. In: Silva- Souza, A.T., Lizama, M.A.P. and Takemoto, R.M. (eds) *Patologia e sanidade de organismos aquáticos.* Massoni, Maringá, Brazil, 404 pp.

Seriani, R., Moreira, L.B., Abessa, D.M.S., Maranho, L.A., Abujamara, L.D. *et al.* (2010a) Hematological analysis of *Micropogonias furnieri* from two estuaries of Baixada Santista, São Paulo, Brazil. *Brazilian Journal of Oceanography* 58, 87–89.

Seriani, R., Ranzani-Paiva, M.J.T., Napoleão, S.R. and Silva-Souza, A.T. (2010b) Hematological characteristics, frequency of micronuclei and nuclear abnormalities in peripheral of fish from São Francisco river Basin, Minas Gerais State, Brazil. *Acta Scientiarum, Biological Sciences* 33(1), 107–112.

Seriani, R., Abessa, D.M.S., Kirschbaum, A.A., Pereira, C.D.S., Ranzani-Paiva, M.J.T. *et al.* (2011) Relationship between water toxicity and hematological changes in *Oreochromis niloticus. Brazilian Journal of Aquatic Science and Technology* 15(2), 47–53.

Seriani, R., Abessa, D.M.S., Kirschbaum, A.A., Pereira, C.D.S., Ranzani-Paiva, M.J.T. *et al.* (2012) Water toxicity and cyto-genotoxicity biomarkers in fish *Oreochromis niloticus* (Cichlidae). *Journal of the Brazilian Society of Ecotoxicology* 7, 79–84.

Shigdar, S., Harford, A., Alister, C. and Ward, A.C. (2009) Cytochemical characterization of the leucocytes and thrombocytes from Murray cod (*Maccullochella peelii peelii*, Mitchell). *Fish & Shellfish Immunology* 26, 731–736.

Silva, W.F., Egami, M.I., Santos, A.A., Antoniazzi, M.M., Silva, M., Gutierre, R.C. and Paiva, M.J.R. (2011) Cytochemical, immunocytochemical and ultrastructural observations on leukocytes and thrombocytes of fat snook (*Centropomus parallelus*). *Fish & Shellfish Immunology* 31, 571–577.

Silva-Souza, A.T., Ranzani-Paiva, M.J.T. and Machado, P.M. (2002) Hematologia: O quadro sangüíneo de peixes do rio Tibagi. In: Medri, M.E., Bianchini, E., Shibatta, O.A. and Pimenta, J.A. (eds) *A bacia do rio Tibagi.* Editora: Edição dos Editores, Londrina, Brazil, pp. 449–471.

Smit, N.J., Eiras, J.C., Ranzani-Paiva, M.J.T. and Davies, A.J. (2002) A *Desseria* sp. from fathead mullet in South Africa. *Journal of Marine Biology and Assessment* 82, 675–676.

Steinhagen, D., Oesterreich, B. and Körting, W. (1997) Carp coccidiosis: Clinical and hematological observations of carp infected with *Goussia carpelli. Diseases of Aquatic Organisms* 30, 137–143.

Sudagara, M., Mohammadizarejabada, A., Mazandarania, R. and Pooralimotlagha, S. (2009) The efficacy of clove powder as an anesthetic and its effects on hematological parameters on roach (*Rutilus rutilus*). *Journal of Aquaculture Feed Science and Nutrition* 1(1), 1–5.

Sweilum, M.A. (2006) Effect of sublethal toxicity of some pesticides on growth parameters, haematological properties and total production of Nile tilapia (*Oreochromis niloticus* L.) and water quality of ponds. *Aquaculture Research* 37, 1079–1089.

Tavares-Dias, M. (2006a) Cytochemical method for staining fish basophils. *Journal of Fish Biology* 69, 312–317.

Tavares-Dias, M. (2006b) A morphological and cytochemical study of erythrocytes, thrombocytes and leukocytes in four freshwater teleosts. *Journal of Fish Biology* 68, 1822–1833.

Tavares-Dias, M. and Barcellos, J.F.M. (2005) Peripheral blood cells of the armored catfish *Hoplosternum littorale* Hancock, 1828: A morphological and cytochemical study. *Brazilian Journal of Morphological Science* 22(4), 215–220.

Tavares-Dias, M. and Moraes, F.R. (2003) Características hematológicas de *Tilapia rendalli* Boulenger, 1896 (Osteichthyes: Cichlidae) capturada em "pesque-pague" de Franca, São Paulo, Brasil. *Bioscience Journal* 19(1), 107–114.

Tavares-Dias, M. and Moraes, F.R. (2004) *Hematologia de peixes teleósteos.* Villimpress, Ribeirão Preto, Brazil, 144 pp.

Tavares-Dias, M., Sandrim, E.F.S. and Campos-Filho, E. (1999) Características hematológicas do tambaqui Colossoma macropomum Cuvier (Osteichthyes, Characidae) em sistema de monocultivo intensivo. II. Leucócitos. *Revista brasileira de Zoologia* 16(1), 175–184.

Tavares-Dias, M., Mataqueiro, M.I. and Perecin, D. (2002) Total leukocyte counts in fishes by direct or indirect methods? *Boletim do Instituto de Pesca* 28(2), 155–161.

Tavares-Dias, M., Moraes, F.R., Onaka, E.M. and Rezende, P.C.B. (2007a) Changes in blood parameters of hybrid tambacu fish parasitized by *Dolops carvalhoi* (Crustacea, Branchiura), a fish louse. *Veterinarski Arhiv* 77, 355–363.

Tavares-Dias, M., Ono, E.A., Pilarski, F. and Moraes, F.R. (2007b) Can thrombocytes participe in the removal of cellular debris in the blood circulation of teleost fish? A cytochemical study and ultrastructural analysis. *Journal of Applie Ichthiology* 23, 709–712.

Tavares-Dias, M., Affonso, E.G., Oliveira, S.R., Marcon, J.L. and Egami, M.I. (2008) Comparative study on hematological parameters of farmed matrinxã, *Brycon amazonicus*, Spix and Agassiz, 1829 (Characidae:Bryconinae) with others Bryconinae species. *Acta Amazônica* 38(4), 799–806.

Tavares-Dias, M., Monteiro, A.M.C., Affonso, E.G. and Amaral, K.D.S. (2011) Weight-length relationship, condition factor and blood parameters of farmed *Cichla temensis* Humboldt, 1821 (Cichlidae) in central Amazon. *Neotropical Ichthyology* 9(1), 113–119.

Tocidlowski, M.E. and Stoskopf, K. (1997) Comparison of sodium polyanetholesulfonate with EDTA and heparin anticoagulants by assessing packed cell volume and blood smear quality of blood from hybrid white bass x striped bass. *Journal of Aquatic Animal Health* 9, 151–155.

Tort, L., Puigcerver, M., Crespo, S. and Padrós, F. (2002) Cortisol and haematological response in sea bream and trout subjected to the anesthetics clove oil and 2-phenoxyethanol. *Aquaculture Research* 33(11), 907–910.

Ueda, I.K., Egami, M.I., Sasso, W.S. and Matushima, E.R. (2001) Cytochemical aspects of the peripheral blood cells of *Oreochromis (Tilapia) niloticus* (Linnaeus, 1758) Cichlidae, Teleostei — Part II. *Brazilian Journal of Veterinary Animal Science* 8, 273–277.

Veiga, M.L., Ranzani-Paiva, M.J.T., Rodrigues, E.L. and Egami, M.I. (2002) Aspectos morfológicos y citoquímicos de las células sanguíneas de *Salminus maxillosus* Valenciennes, 1840 (Characiformes, Characidae). *Revista Chilena de Anatomia* 18(2), 245–250.

Velišek, J., Svobodová, Z. and Piačková, V. (2007a) Effects of 2-Phenoxyethanol anaesthesia on haematological profile on common carp (*Cyprinus carpio*) and rainbow trout (*Oncorhynchus mykiss*). *Acta Veterinaria Brno* 76(3), 487–492.

Velišek, J., Wlasow, T., Gomulka, P., Svobodova, Z. and Novotny, L. (2007b) Efects of 2-phenoxyethanol anaesthesia on sheatfsh (*Silurus glanis* L.). *Veterinary Medicine* 52(3), 103–110.

Wang, K., Zhuang, T., Su, Z., Chi, M. and Wang, H. (2021) Antibiotic residues in wastewaters from sewage treatment plants and pharmaceutical industries: Occurrence, removal and environmental impacts. *Science of The Total Environment* 788, 147811.

Wagner, G.M., Lubin, B.H. and Chiu, D.T.Y. (1988) Oxidative damage to red blood cells. In: Chow, C.K. (ed.) *Cellular Antioxidant Defense Mechanisms*. CRC Press, Boca Raton, Florida.

Waldmann-Meyer, H. and Schilling, K. (1956) The interaction of bromophenol blue with serum albumin and γ-globulin in acid medium. *Archives of Biochemistry and Biophysics* 64(2), 291–301.

Walencik, J. and Witeska, M. (2007) The effects of anticoagulants on hematological indices and blood cell morphology of common carp (*Cyprinus carpio* L.). *Comparative Biochemistry and Physiology: Part C: Toxicology and Pharmacology* 146(3), 331–335.

Walencik, J. and Witeska, M. (2011) Disodium EDTA used as anticoagulant causes hemolysis in common carp blood. *Turkish Journal of Veterinary and Animal Science* 35(1), 1–6.

Wintrobe, M.M. (1934) Variations in the size and hemoglobin content of erythrocytes in the blood of various vertebrates. *Folia Haematologica* 51, 32–49.

Yu, J.H., Han, J.J. and Park, S.W. (2010) Haematological and biochemical alterations in Korean catfish, *Silurus asotus*, experimentally infected with *Edwardsiella tarda*. *Aquaculture Research* 41, 295–302.

Annex 1

Manual for using automatic micropipettes

1. To pipette blood (and other liquids denser than water), it is better to press the button up to second stop.
2. Hold the pipette vertically, and place the tip in the blood, but not too deep.
3. Release the button slowly and steadily to aspirate the blood.
4. Wait 1 or 2 s before drawing the tip away from the blood. Wipe the outside of the tip with a moist tissue, without touching the tip.
5. Place the end of the tip on the inside wall of the receptacle at a 10-40° angle.
6. Press the button continuously up to the first stop, and wait 1 s.
7. Hold the button down at the first stop, and withdraw the pipette from the receptacle keeping the tip against wall of the receptacle.
8. Release the button, and discard the tip pressing on the ejector button. Only it is necessary to change the tip if the liquid to be aspirated is changed.
9. When a liquid denser and more viscous than water is dispensed, additionally wait for 1 or 2 s at the end of the first stage before eliminating the liquid.

Index

Absolute polycythemia, 27
Acanthocytes, 27
Acid phosphatase, 54, 56–57, 59–60
Adaptive strategies, 2
Alkaline phosphatase, 54, 56–58
Anachromasia, 27
Anemia, 22, 23
  cause of, 25–26
  classification, 26–27
Anesthetics, 4, 5
Anisocytosis, 26
Arterial bulb, 7
Auricle/atrium, 7
Automatic pipettes, 15, 16

Basophils, 41, 43, 68
Benzocaine, 5–6, 9, 10
Blood cells, 14, 34
  basophils, 41, 43
  eosinophils, 40–42
  erythrocytes, 35, 36, 50
  heterophils, 39–41
  immature leukocytes, 41, 44
  lymphocytes, 36–38
  monocytes, 35, 37
  neutrophils, 38–40
  PAS-positive granular leukocyte, 37, 39
  thrombocytes, 42, 45
Blood count method, 2
Blood layers, 15
Blood loss, 25
Blood sampling, fish
  anticoagulants, 6–7
  blood vessels puncture, 7, 9–10
  capture, 4, 5

cardiac puncture, 10, 12
circulatory system, 7, 8
confinement, 4–6
gill puncture, 10–12
intracardiac puncture, 10, 11
storage, 12–13
techniques, 3
Blood tests, 3
Bromophenol blue method, 61–62, 66, 67

Carbohydrate, 52
Centrifugation time, 21
Chlorobutanol, 4–5
Citrates, 6
Clinical hematology, 1
  blood, 2
  challenges, 1
  circulatory system, 1–2
  in fish production systems, 3
  nutritional requirement evaluation, 1
  techniques, 3
Clove oil, 4, 5, 6
Cloves, powdered, 5
Cyanmethemoglobin reagent, 22–23
Cytochemical methods, 51–52
  acid phosphatase, 56–57, 59–60
  alkaline phosphatase, 54, 56–58
  bromophenol blue method, 61–62, 66, 67
  leukocyte cytoplasm, blue precipitate in, 60
  metachromatic staining, 62–64, 67, 68
  napthyl AS-D acetate, 59–60, 63–65
  periodic acid-Schiff method, 51–55
  peroxidase, 57, 61, 63
  phosphatases, 52–54
  Sudan Black B method, 60–61, 66

Defective erythropoiesis, 25
Differential white blood cells, 32–34
Dilution, 15, 16, 18

EDTA, 6, 7
Endogenous conditions, 2
Eosinophilic peroxidase (EPO), 59
Eosinophils, 40–42
Error, causes of, 19, 21, 32
Erythremia, 27
Erythroblasts, 34
Erythrocytes, 14, 15, 35, 36, 50
        accelerated destruction, 26
        counting, 18
        with insufficient hemoglobin, 26
Erythrocytosis, 27
Erythrogram, 14
        anemia, 25–27
        blood layers, 14, 15
        red blood cell counting, 14–20
                dilution, 20, 22
                hematocrit, 20–22, 24–26
                hemoglobin level, 22–23, 26
                mean corpuscular hemoglobin
                        concentration (MCHC), 23
                mean corpuscular volume (MCV), 23
                number, 19
                procedure, 17, 19, 23, 24
                RBC indices, 23–25
Etiological anemias, 27
Eugenol, 5
Exogenous conditions, 2

Fish blood constituents, 2
Fish heart, 7
Formol-citrate, 17

Giemsa method, 31
Glycogen, 52

Hayem's solution, 17, 20
Hematocrit, 20–22, 24–26
Hematological changes, 6
Hemoglobin level, 22–23, 26
Hemogram
        blood smear, staining of, 29–32
        erythroblasts counting, 34
        erythrogram (see Erythrogram)
        thrombocyte count (THRC), 28–29, 34
        white blood cells count, 32
                differential, 32–34
                interpretation, 34, 35
        white blood count (WBC), 28–29
Hemogregarines, 42, 46
Hemoparasites, 48–49

Heparin, 6, 7
Heterophils, 39–41
Hypochromic anemia, 27
Hypoxia, 23

Immature erythrocytes, 34
Immature leukocytes, 41, 44

Leukocytes, 18, 34, 51, 60
Lymphocytes, 36–38

Macrocytic anemia, 26
May-Grünwald-Giemsa (MGG) stain, 31
Mean corpuscular hemoglobin concentration
        (MCHC), 23
Mean corpuscular volume (MCV), 23
Megaloblastic anemia, 26
Menthol, 4, 6
Metachromasia, 62, 64
Metachromatic staining, 62–64, 67, 68
Microcytic anemia, 26
Microhematocrit, 21
Monocytes, 35, 37
Morphological anemias, 27
MS 222, 4
Myeloperoxidase detection, 57, 61, 63
Myxosporids, 47

Na_2EDTA, 6
Naphthol AS-D acetate (NASDA) esterase, 60
Napthyl AS-D acetate, 59–60, 63–65
Neubauer chamber, 15, 17, 18
Neutrophils, 38–40
Normochromic anemia, 27
Normocytic anemia, 26

Oxalates, 6

Parasites, 42–44, 46–50
PAS-positive granular leukocyte, 37, 39
Periodic acid-Schiff method, 51–55
Peroxidase, 57, 61, 63
2-phenoxyethanol, 4, 5
Phosphatases, 52–54
Poikilocytes, 26
Polychromasia, 27
Polycythemia, 27
Polypropylene Eppendorf microtubes, 12, 13
Protozoan trypanosomes, 42, 46

RBC clearance, 26, 27
Red blood cell counting, 14–20

dilution, 20, 22
hematocrit, 20–22, 24–26
hemoglobin level, 22–23, 26
mean corpuscular hemoglobin concentration
    (MCHC), 23
mean corpuscular volume (MCV), 23
number, 19
procedure, 17, 19, 23, 24
RBC indices, 23–25
Relative polycythemia, 27
Rickettsiae, 42, 46

Saline, 17
Smears, 28–32, 64
Sodium citrate, 6
Sodium heparin, 6
Sodium polyanethole sulfonate, 6
Spherocytes, 26

Staining, 28–32
Sudan Black B method, 60–61, 66

Thoma pipette, 14, 15
Thrombocyte count (THRC), 28–29, 34
Thrombocytes, 42, 45
Toluidine-hydrogen peroxide method, 54, 61, 62
Total plasma protein (TPP), 21
Transitory polycythemia, 27

Venous sinus, 7
Ventricle, 7
Visual method, 15

White blood cells (WBC), 14–16
White blood count (WBC), 28–29

www.ingramcontent.com/pod-product-compliance
Lightning Source LLC
Chambersburg PA
CBHW040136200326
41458CB00025B/6283